Ramshackle Glam

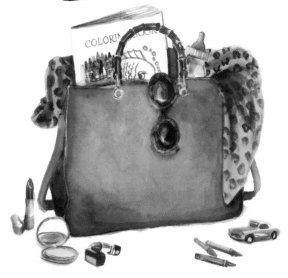

THE NEW MOM'S HAPHAZARD GUIDE TO (Almost) HAVING IT ALL

Jordan Reid

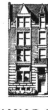

Running Press
PHILADELPHIA · LONDON

ISBN 978-0-7624-5304-7
Library of Congress Control Number: 2013955296

E-book ISBN 978-0-7624-5305-4

9 8 7 6 5 4 3 2 1
Digit on the right indicates the number of this printing

Edited by Cindy De La Hoz
Designed by Amanda Richmond
Ramshackle Glam logo design by Naava Katz
Typography: Mrs. Eaves, Gotham, and Tamarillo

Running Press Book Publishers
2300 Chestnut Street
Philadelphia, PA 19103-4371

Visit us on the web!
www.runningpress.com

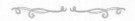

For Kendrick, who makes everything possible.

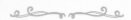

Contents

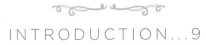

BEAUTY
(Your Hair Is Awesome, and That's a Good Start)

HOME
(Babies Throw Up a Lot, But You Still Probably Need to Own a Couch)

EASY RECIPES
FOR BABY AND YOU
(Go Buy a Slow Cooker Right Now)

THE TOUGH STUFF
(Let's All Screw Up Together)

GETTING OUT

(Your Baby Is Amazing and Super Cute,
But Not Everyone in the World Is
Going to Agree With You on That One)

Conclusion

"The only true currency in this bankrupt world . . .
is what we share with someone else when we're uncool."

—LESTER BANGS

(*Almost Famous*)

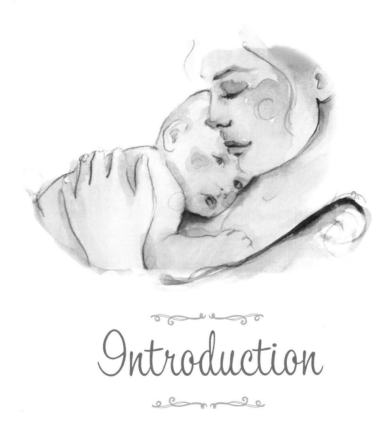

Introduction

About three months after I found out I was pregnant, I went to a dinner party at my friend Morgan's house. Another woman there had her one-month-old baby with her, and upon finding out I was expecting immediately insisted I hold the child "for practice."

In my experience, you know what happens when you hold other people's babies? They cry horrible, soul-wrenching tears, and make you feel extremely guilty. And then you hand them back to their mom and they immediately become happy again, and it becomes clear to all present that you have terrible parental instincts and should never be allowed to come into contact with children, ever.

I did not want to hold this baby.

But I did anyway, mostly because I didn't want to insult the nice woman who was offering me her infant. I bundled his delicate little body into my arms, no idea which part of him was supposed to go where or how I would keep his head from falling right off of his neck, and then decided that sitting would be my best bet. I set him down on my lap and held on to his arms like they were teeny-tiny life preservers, hoping desperately that he wouldn't make any sudden moves or wail piteously, having gathered that the woman holding him was not only not his mother, but also quite clearly not a particularly maternal person.

He looked up at me, and I looked down at him. We evaluated each other. But—to my considerable surprise—he didn't make a peep. He looked . . . pretty much okay, actually. It was the first time that I thought maybe—just maybe—I might be able to do this "mom" thing.

A few months later, my son was born and I realized that I was right: Not only "can" I do it . . . I *love* doing it.

If you're a new mom (and if you're reading a book with "New Mom" right there in the title there's a decent chance that you are), enormous congratulations to you. You made it through childbirth—a thing that no human being in possession of pain receptors and the potential for hormonal fluctuations should be able to make it through—and came out on the other side with a brand-new life, made richer by your tiny, wrinkly addition in ways that you expected and in ways you never dreamed.

New motherhood is awesome.

You know what's not awesome? That you're about to hear these words a lot (a weird-lot. An all-the-time-from-every-single-person-you-pass-on-the-street-lot):

"Oh, it goes *so* fast. Enjoy every second!"

My son is nearly two now, and is walking (or rather sprinting, primarily toward things like swimming pools and stairways) and talking (or, more accurately, using the word *no* as a placeholder for the entirety of the English language, including the word *yes*) and becoming more and more his own person with each passing moment. Having abandoned the wilderness of the Newborn Era for the shores of Toddlerhood, I can vouch for the fact that this whole parenting thing is really fun, and gets even more fun every single day as your child learns more and more ways to interact with the world around him.

And as annoying as all that enjoy-every-second-ness was (oh my god, super annoying, and guaranteed to make me terrified that I'm not savoring every! single! moment! *enough*), I'm starting to see what these people meant . . . because now that my son is in the midst of the second year of his life, time is sprinting by at light speed, and all I want to do is stop the clocks so that I can spend more hours watching him wobbling all over the house and trying to destroy things. These days, he *is* growing up too fast.

The first year, though? That took *forever*.

Seriously, I look at pictures from when my son was six months old, and they feel like they were taken sometime back in 1983.

Why is this?

Because time passes really, *reallllllllly* slowly when you're not sleeping. And when about 80 percent of your way-too-many waking hours are spent bouncing a very small (yet surprisingly heavy) person up and down while emitting an extremely loud whooshing noise directly into his eardrum because that is the only thing—literally the only thing—that will stop him from crying . . . nonstop . . . for about seven months.

I remember once, around 4:30 a.m., I was doing cartwheels or whatever it was that I had to do to calm our child down out in the living room, and my husband, Kendrick, came wandering out to see if I was okay. I looked up at him all wild-eyed, and all of the sudden saw myself through his eyes: a crazy lady with hair that was basically in a mohawk, wearing one of those robes that are cozy but that you really don't want people to see you in—for the third day straight—with a rivulet of spit-up running down one shoulder. It's also pretty likely that the robe was hanging open and that I was still attached to a breast pump. For those of you who have never seen a breast pump, let me be clear: This is not a sexy thing.

I mean, look: It's completely normal to be a total disaster in the weeks (months) after childbirth, and I'd heard that this was how those first few weeks (months) were probably going to go . . . but it still threw me for a loop. I suppose that deep down I pictured myself as a glowing little postpartum Mother Teresa, all joy and benevolence and blissful calm. I certainly never pictured myself pacing our living room floor while doing my very best impersonation of an angry water buffalo having a bad hair day.

In case I haven't yet made this clear: I didn't really handle the first few weeks following the birth of our son all too well. I felt scared, and overwhelmed, and lonely, and I worried constantly about whether we had created a safe and comfortable environment for our new arrival in our fourth-floor walk-up apartment, conveniently located smack in the center of a construction zone on New York City's Upper East Side. And part of it was hormones, and part of it was just the way it goes, but part of it was also that when I stepped back for a moment, I had trouble even recognizing myself when I looked in the mirror.

I am someone who loves—cherishes, even—the little luxuries in life. I started an entire website, Ramshackle Glam, devoted to the idea that these small joys are not just wonderful . . . they're *important*, and they're worth taking the time to integrate into your world in whatever way makes sense for you. I don't mean Chanel dresses and limo rides to eight-course meals at four-star restaurants; I mean a nice candle that smells like cucumbers, or a beautiful handbag that actually fits everything you need it to fit and looks even better with age, or watching a truly atrocious horror movie (because those are the best kind) while drinking a big glass of wine . . . and, yeah, a little mascara and lip gloss, if that's what makes you feel good.

Let's get one thing straight, right off the bat: Having a baby changes your life. A lot. And that's good and okay and the way that it should be, because the baby is the Number One Priority. You don't need me to tell you that. But something that my first year of motherhood taught me is that it's important to remember to make yourself a little bit of a priority as well—to carve out slices of life that aren't about your significant other, or about your baby, or about what others want from you . . . but are rather about *you*.

There are plenty of books out there about how to take care of a baby, or books about how to diet and work out after giving birth. This book isn't a replacement for those guides; it's simply an addition. In these pages, you'll find information on all those things you kind of want to know but aren't quite sure who to ask about . . . like how to dress to celebrate (or downplay) the new shape that you've developed courtesy of breast-feeding, or how to rearrange your living room so it doesn't attack your child but still looks respectably chic, or how to do your makeup in five minutes flat with one hand while keeping that bouncy chair going with the other.

The little luxuries that you maintain in your life can be faster than they used to be, sure. And they'll certainly involve more corner-cutting, but that's okay; the point is that they're *there*. There to make you feel like yourself, to make you feel like an adult, and even to make you feel . . .yes . . . a little glam.

This book isn't about being Superwoman—oh my god, no. It's about finding realistic ways to enjoy the amazing new addition to your life while still maintaining a semblance of your spectacular self. Life changes, families expand, and people evolve to fill the corners of their new lives, and that's a great thing. . . .

But it's also important to remember that it's okay to take a second every once in awhile to paint your nails purple just because you love the color.

Because *that's* cool.

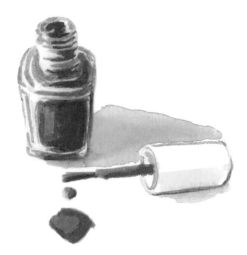

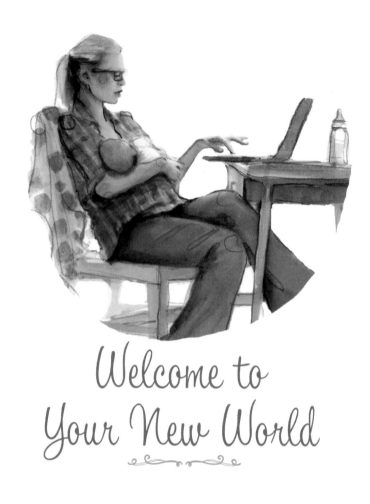

Welcome to Your New World

It's Okay to Be a Nut for a While

I don't remember a whole lot of what went on in the hours following the birth of my son, mostly because I was on lots and lots of drugs.

I do recall putting on mascara because (a) I'm vain, sue me, and (b) for whatever reason our society has decided that a woman who has just spent several hours sweating and screaming should be confronted with permanent, high-definition evidence of what, exactly, several hours of sweating and screaming look like on her face. And then that evidence should go on Facebook, where people like distant relatives and ex-boyfriends can see it.

What I do remember: falling asleep in a room no bigger than a closet while the sun came up, my hour-old baby curled on my chest with his wrinkly little hand tucked under his chin. I remember watching my husband hovering over the bassinet, silent, breathing along with our son and looking flat-out amazed at what he had created. I also remember that for whatever reason (good ones involving tests and other hospital-y things, I'm sure), the nurses were constantly wheeling my baby away into other rooms for varying amounts of time. And while that made me sort of nervous every time it happened, it also kind of made me feel like, you know . . .

Whew.

Because then I had a second to drink my hospital-issue apple juice, or make my twenty-minute round-trip journey to the bathroom, or just not be all "Holy shit, that is an effing *person* who used to be in and is now out, and in approximately thirty hours he is going to come live in my fourth-floor walk-up apartment with my insane dogs and slanty floors and dust bunnies. And he doesn't even have a *functional belly button*." (Not that belly buttons function, but if they did, a newborn's belly button would really not be taking care of business. That is a bad situation, right there.)

I don't care who you are. Even if you have nannies and fully furnished Pottery Barn nurseries coming out your eyeballs, taking a baby home for the very first time is a scary thing.

And so when the sun went down on that first night and a lovely, smiling woman came by to ask me whether I would like her to take my newborn to the nursery so that I could get some for-real rest, I took the advice of every single parenting book and actual parent that I'd consulted prior to delivery, and gave her an enthusiastic, "Yes ma'am, thank you." Away he went, all bundled up and cute, and apparently I passed out.

But then half an hour later there I was, lurching up from my hospital bed like the zombie version of the Creature from the Black Lagoon, stumbling into the hallway barefoot and sweaty with my maternity underwear butt out and about for all to see. I was in a total panic, picturing my tiny, fragile, sweet baby boy all alone in a plastic cube in the middle of a vast room, terrified and wanting his mama and probably developing irreparable abandonment issues *right that very minute*.

And so I did what any logical person would do: charged toward the nurses' station like a rampaging elephant, shrieking something along the lines of "GIVE ME MY BABY." It may have been those exact words, said in exactly those capital letters. Don't forget about the smooshy mascara, druggy eyes, and maternity butt. Those are important details; I want to make sure that you get the full picture here.

The nurses looked at me as if I had just strolled up, announced that I was Barbra Streisand, and burst into a hearty rendition of "Don't Rain on My Parade." They sat in stunned silence for a moment, staring at the thing that may or may not be trying to tackle them (me). They assessed.

And then:

". . . Would you like your child, ma'am?"

"YES PLEASE GIVE ME MY BABY."

"Okay."

Here's a stunner: They don't actually kidnap your child when they take him to the nursery so you can sleep. He's yours, and you get to have him if you want him. That concept had escaped me for the time being, though . . . and was the first indicator that things were going to be slightly whooey in Whoville for a while.

A quick sampling of events that transpired over the next two weeks or so:

• What I recall as a major medical incident right in the middle of the crosswalk on Park Avenue, but which my husband refers to as my Drama Queen Swoon Moment.

• An altercation with a CVS pharmaceutical attendant who needed to give me my pain medication prescription *right now*, and whom I alerted to that fact with a second bout of dramatic swooning followed in rapid succession by yelling.

- A subsequent incident involving the aforementioned CVS pharmaceutical attendant during which he reportedly informed my husband that he needed to "control his woman."
- A hysterical crying attack for no reason at all that literally frightened away a woman outside the hospital who had stopped to compliment me on my newborn. (Her: "Oh, what a beautiful little—" Me: "WAAAAAA.")
- A hysterical crying attack because our friends brought us a home-cooked meal on our first night back from the hospital, and it was nice of them.
- A hysterical crying attack because *Where the Wild Things Are* fell off the shelf, making me realize how completely unprepared I was for even the most basic tasks associated with motherhood.
- A hysterical crying attack because ASPCA ads with Sarah McLachlan songs exist. (I continue to think this one makes sense.)

The fact that my husband didn't go fleeing into the night carrying only his Brand-New Dad Cigar is a mini-miracle. But he didn't, and we got through it and came out the other side, and what all this taught me is that giving birth is not—surprise, surprise—anything approaching a small deal. It's not just your life that's thrown into upheaval for a while . . . it's your *self*. Your body. Even your mind, sometimes.

And you know what? That's okay. When every single part of you goes through a tectonic shift, you're allowed to act a little nutty for a minute. Just do your best to roll with it, take your time, reach out for help if help is what you need. . . .

And tell your partner to catch you when you swoon. Even if they think you're faking. It's their job.

Mom, I'm Home!

You know those grandparents who swear up and down that they brought their new-borns home from the hospital and stowed them away in, like, a shoebox next to the Victrola or something?

You know the type:

[*World-weary, gravelly voice*]: "I didn't need any of these schmancy *bassinets* back when I had [*weirdly childlike variant on name of person who is presently an adult*]. We just pulled some clothing out of a dresser drawer, called it a crib, and got on with business."

While I think that pretty much every single one of the grandparents who says something like this is lying (or, come on, at least *embellishing*) they do have a point. And the point is this: a newborn doesn't need a whole lot. For the first couple of months, they actually don't really need much of anything.

But hold on a second! Be careful not to get all impressed by my levelheaded wisdom and down-to-earth-ness here, because even though I understood this point on a surface level when I was pregnant, oh my goodness did it ever take its time coming in for a wheels-down landing in my brain. Going into this whole deal, of course I knew that having a child wasn't about having "things," but still: part of me thought that if my baby was going to survive the first year of his life in anything approaching a happy, comfortable state I was for sure going to have to find a way to fit every single gadget and gizmo and bottle warmer stopper changer wiper thing on the market into our very (very) small apartment. Except I didn't know what any of these things were, or which ones one I should buy, or how I might go about using them.

And so I sort of lost it.

I Cried in Babies 'R' Us

The thing about being the very first of your friends to get pregnant is this:

1. Very, very few of them want to talk about babies (I don't blame them; I'm pregnant and I don't particularly want to talk about babies either . . . except I sort of have to, because I have never, ever been around an infant and have a bit to learn); and

2. There's no one to give you "Oh, I just went through that"–style advice.

My mom is amazing, but it's been awhile since she did this, and we're both sort of equally perplexed by the sheer volume of options out there for everything from cribs to toys to breast milk storage bags (do those go directly into the bottle? Or do you pour the milk out of them and into the bottle once they're defrosted? And why will no one give me a straight answer on this?).

What I need is a friend who has gone through this recently to walk through Babies "R" Us with me and tell me that I am not already a failure as a mother because I don't have room for/can't afford a bouncy seat, a swing, a play yard, and a floor mobile thingy (the gentleman in the store already sent me into a meltdown by telling me that a wide variety of play areas is crucial for early motor-skill development).

I want her to tell me when to go for cute and fun, and when to go for practical. I want to know if there's a sling out there that is sturdy but doesn't cover up your whole body.

And I want her to help me figure out exactly what A Day in the Life is going to look like a few months from now, because I can't picture it, and I work out of the house by myself all day long with a hundred stairs between me and the rest of the world, and no dishwasher or washing machine, and two little dogs that need walking and think that every single fluffy thing that moseys through the door is a toy special-ordered just for them, and I don't know how I'm going to do it. I mean, I'm obviously *going* to do it—that I'm sure of—but I'd just like to have some idea how. In advance.

And so I cried in Babies "R" Us. It was when the salesman was telling me that pretty much every stroller that has the features I'm looking for weighs upward of eighteen pounds, which I'm not certain is a possible weight for me to lift (plus baby, plus associated bags and accessories) up and down four flights of steps every day.

Do I sound like I'm complaining? I really don't mean to. I very much want this—I've wanted it my whole life, more than anything—and am so grateful. I've always been scared that I wouldn't be able to get pregnant, and the fact that I am . . . I'm aware that it's the greatest, most incredible gift in the world. I know that it's not about things, and that babies need much less than you think they do (or than stores will have you think they do). I also get that I'm not in the worst situation in the world—far from it—and that in fact I'm very lucky to have the things that I do (which, most importantly, include a supportive family and group of friends). And of course the answer is that I'll figure it all out, and that it'll be fine . . . better than fine. Wonderful. I know that.

I just want to do this really, really well. I want to pay attention to every moment, because another thing that I know is that it goes very, very fast, and that you miss it when it's over. That's all.

As it turns out, I was right about several things: Pregnancy is an incredible gift, I was not in the worst situation in the world, and I would figure it out (and it would be fine). I was also, alas, right about the stroller situation: I went for the lightest one I could find, and it was misery from the first day I lugged that thing up those four flights until the day we moved. But when it comes to the rest of it . . . eh. I could really just have relaxed a bit.

Because the truth is, you don't need the half of it.

The stuff? Oh, the stuff comes *later*, when your child is doing things like moving more than an inch in any one direction. Enjoy the relative lack of clutter while you have it, and stick to the basics.

NEW MAMA MUST-HAVES

BREASTFEEDING PILLOW. But! But but but. Do not go out and spend eighty dollars on a fancy-pants cushion for your wee one's head; any old firm-ish pillow will do the trick nicely. And if you're even a tiny bit handy, you can do what I did and DIY your very own custom-made breastfeeding pillow out of that full-body pillow that you snuggled up with while you were pregnant. Just snip it in half at its narrowest point, tie off the ends, and use whichever half feels more comfortable.

SO, SO MANY BURP CLOTHS. During a trip to a baby stuff store when I was nine months pregnant, I tried to buy an adorable fifteen-dollar burp cloth. Unfortunately I was with my mother, and so my desire for a quilted square trimmed in silk and covered with tiny blue elephants was summarily dismissed. Instead, she handed me a bulk package of sadly unpatterned white burp cloths, insisting that it didn't matter if they were cute . . . it mattered if they were plentiful.

I wanted elephants. She wanted me to be a reasonable human being. And of course she was right, because mothers are always right (a fact that used to be annoying but is now awesome, considering that I am now a mother and can announce "Mothers are always right" whenever my husband disagrees with me on any point at all, including whether or not I should buy that dress I saw at Anthropologie). Buy your burp cloths cheap, and then buy more of them than you think you need. I went through an average of ten a day for many, many months . . . and if you constantly have one draped across your shoulder or whatever surface the baby is laying on you'll save yourself a ton of time cleaning things like grown-up clothing, play mats, upholstery, and your hair.

DIAPERS. Obviously. But try to resist the urge to stock up on the newborn size—your baby will grow quickly and in unpredictable bursts, so in those first few weeks diapers should really be a buy-as-needed situation.

A DECENT BREAST PUMP. I went budget on mine. This was a mistake, because pumping one side at a time is not only an enormous pain . . . it's enormously time-consuming. I ended up spending practically every second that my son was asleep desperately trying to fill my refrigerator with enough supplies to keep him going during the times when I had to leave him with my husband or a sitter . . . and since my pump required me to sit down and physically hold it in place, that meant that the only things I could accomplish during those precious naps were tasks requiring one hand and no movement whatsoever. (I wrote a lot of extremely short, typo-ridden emails during this period.) Go for a hands-free electric version that pumps both sides at once. They're expensive, but in my opinion they're completely worth it.

SWADDLING BLANKETS. Here's another example of where to save your money. My favorite swaddling blanket ended up being a plain pale-blue one simply because it was the right size and thickness, was machine-washable, and didn't sass me when I tried to tuck it around my son. I'm also partial to the blankets that come pre-affixed with Velcro patches; they streamline the whole process enormously.

A CHAIR FOR YOU. I think a cozy rocker is a really nice thing to have when you're sitting in a dark room nursing a baby at three o'clock in the morning. If you're going to splurge, just be sure to go for a chair that won't look out of place in your home if you want to move it out of the nursery later on. (In other words, maybe go for a chic style in a neutral color over one covered in pictures of baby sheep.)

A CHAIR FOR BABY. Just a fact: You need a safe place to put your baby on those occasions when you're forced to use both of your hands for something else. That can be a towel spread on the floor, an actual play mat with toys dangling overhead . . . or my own personal pick: a chair that both vibrates and swings, so you can be sure that whichever motion is your own little grumper's preference, that's the motion he gets.

EASY EDIBLES. During the first couple of weeks that my son was home, I subsisted almost entirely on things that I could eat with one hand, without sitting down. There were no plates. No utensils. No leafy greens gently sautéed in olive oil and sprinkled with flaxseed and ambrosia. This was obviously not a nutritionally ideal situation, but sometimes life gets in the way of your ability to prepare perfectly proportioned meals that hit all the major food groups. Make sure to keep some easy-to-eat things like protein bars and individually wrapped cheeses on hand for "I'm starving and my baby won't let me put him down for even one second" emergencies.

One thing I *insist* you own: a noise machine. One of my best friends, Katie, has two of the most perfect children you've ever met. They're cute, well-behaved, and smart, and when we go out to lunch with her and her kids, once in awhile the younger one will suddenly go all quiet, and it turns out that—oopsie!—he fell asleep, right there in his carrier.

How adorable.

This, just so we're clear, is not a species of child that I recognize from my own gene pool. I like to think that my son is also cute and well-behaved and smart . . . but the sleeping thing? No comprendo. For the first seven or so months of my son's life, you see, in order to get him to even *nap*—forget about actual "sleeping"—I had to jump up and down while saying "SSH! SSH! SSH!" at the top of my lungs (if you can picture the word *ssh* being said at the top of one's lungs, that's what I was doing. I looked like an absolute lunatic).

Anyway, that's where the noise machine came in, and it was the best thing ever, and now I'm obsessed. Even though my son now sleeps through the night I continue to use one in his room because it also helps him sleep through what happens to my dogs when the Chinese food delivery guy comes to the door (or when a neighbor walks past our house or a leaf falls in our backyard or, god forbid, a chipmunk dares to saunter on by), which is that they lose their minds, loudly (*see:* Chapter 4, page 100: "Oh My God, Your Dogs Are Going to Make You So Angry"). I also have a second noise machine installed in our bedroom, because I love it.

Get one. You will love it, too.

(And just so you know, there's no need to buy an *actual* noise machine; if you have a computer stationed reasonably close to the crib you can log onto one of the many free websites that provide twenty-four-hour streaming white noise. Thank me later; what I want you to do right now is go turn the thing on and let you and your infant be lulled to sleep by the gentle sounds of screeching swamp frogs.)

POST-BABY PRESCRIPTION

FORGET ABOUT THE CLOCK. Seriously, forget that it even exists. It does no one any good if you're busy working yourself into a state over whether it's four in the afternoon or four in the morning; until you and your baby figure out a schedule (which may be several weeks—or even months—from now), do your best to go with the flow. I know how hard this can be, especially if you've got other responsibilities to deal with during the day . . . but I promise, it won't last forever. You can do it.

DON'T TRY TO BE SUPERMOM. If ordering in is not your thing and you want to cook, go for simple, quick recipes (see Chapter 5 for some of my favorites). Leave the dishes in the sink overnight. Wear the same T-shirt you wore to bed to run errands the next morning. And don't worry: The fact that things are a little out-of-control right now doesn't mean that you have undergone some fundamental shift and will never again return to being any semblance of an on-top-of-things human being. It'll all come back. *You'll* come back.

BE COZY. The first couple of weeks home with a new baby is a good time for oversized flannel shirts, pajama pants, lip balm, and not a whole lot else. Make comfort a priority, and let your new family live in a little cocoon for a while if that's what makes you happy.

THAT SAID, DON'T STRESS ABOUT "ENJOYING" YOURSELF. You may be one of those people who's all blissed-out postbirth, you may be suffering from hormonal complications, or even depression (in which case don't be afraid to ask for help), or you may just be straight-up freaking out a bit. All of these things are okay. Don't let the people yelling at you to "relish every moment!" upset you; trust me, you'll have plenty of moments to relish later—when you're sleeping for longer than an hour at a stretch.

IF YOU WANT, IGNORE THE TO-DO LISTS THAT EVERYONE AND THEIR MOTHER SENDS YOU, INCLUDING THIS ONE. This is your baby, your life, and your deal, so do what works for *you*.

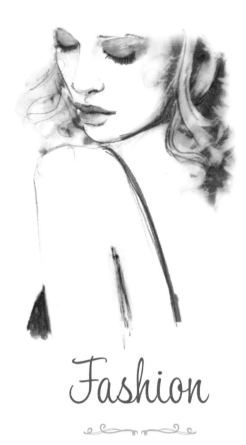

Fashion

❦

(People Have a Whole Lot of Opinions About What You're Wearing, and They Are Going to Tell You What They Are)

Get Your Glitter Eye Shadow On If You Want To

When I was twelve years old, my best friend Arielle and I decided that it was the height of style to go to school every day dressed in old men's striped pajamas that we had scored for $1.50 from the Salvation Army down the street from my apartment. We accessorized the look with lips painted shimmery-white and outlined with dark-brown liner, and then used black kohl pencils to draw enormous snail-shell swirls that extended from the outer corners of our eyes onto our temples. And then we topped it all off with a generous dusting of glitter across those swirls, in addition to our browbones, cheeks, lips . . . wherever we were feeling it on that particular day.

It was quite a look.

We *loved* it.

One afternoon, I had just arrived home from school and was settling in to do a little homework when it suddenly occurred to me that I'd like to try out a self-tanning lotion that I'd seen advertised in *YM*. It was February, I had made my annual transformation into Casper the Friendly Ghost, and I had five bucks burning a hole in my pocket. And so my pajama-ed, be-glittered self decided that a quick run to the drugstore was in order.

Did I bring a coat? I did not! My mother was very pro-coat-in-the-wintertime, as mothers tend to be, and I was in the middle of a pain-in-the-ass stage. So out onto the very cold street I went.

I grew up in Hell's Kitchen, the New York City neighborhood that used to be a hub of Irish and Italian mafia activity (you've seen the place in everything from *Sleepers* to *West Side Story*), but by the time I was born had abandoned those grand, storied roots in favor of being just a straight-up Not-Great Neighborhood. Later, of course, Mayor Giuliani came in and Disney-fied the place (with a mixed bag of responses from residents, some of whom were happy to see all that graffiti get painted over, and others who couldn't stand the idea of Starbucks moving into the stores vacated by mom-and-pop owners who we all knew by name), and now it's all very expensive and fancy . . . but in the years I spent growing up on West 46th Street, it was the kind of neighborhood that attracted lots and lots of people with no place to go.

Around the time I hit puberty, I started being allowed to walk the avenue between the bus stop and our apartment by myself. Any further than that, and chances were I had to find myself an escort of the over-eighteen sort. Conveniently, however, I'm drawing a blank on the "asking my mom for permission to wander our neighborhood alone" part of this particular story.

All right . . . I *may* have skipped that bit. But it was an emergency! I was a girl in need of self-tanner, and I had a major crush on a guy at school who just about exactly resembled Jordan Catalano in *My So-Called Life* (complete with floppy brown hair and a tendency to lean emotionally against lockers), and that is a desperate situation if I've ever heard one. One problem: The closest drugstore was the one inside the Port Authority, which, if you're unfamiliar with the place, was (and continues to be) New York City's primary bus station. Bus stations aren't usually fantastically lovely places in general, and the Port Authority—especially in the early 1990s—was pretty much the opposite of a place where you commonly saw young ladies taking a leisurely stroll around.

When the two plainclothes police officers stationed at the Eighth Avenue entrance to the Port Authority looked up, what they saw run by them was a very cold-looking preteen wearing pajamas and glitter makeup. And probably looking frantic, because, like I said: self-tanner emergency.

So I found myself in the back of a police car, being interrogated by cops who were positive that I was a runaway. (The fact that I tend to immediately burst into tears when confronted by an authority figure surely didn't help matters.)

A few phone calls later, the whole mess was cleared up and I was allowed to return to my apartment (still, alas, *sans* self-tanner). Mom was mad; Jordan Catalano made out with me one afternoon a couple of years later on a brownstone stoop around the corner from school and then graduated, never to be heard from again. So it goes.

The point of this is not to say that this was a particularly smart choice on my part. It wasn't; kids, wear your coats when you go outside in February, please. And it's not even to say that the pajamas were an excellent look for me. They weren't; I abandoned them a couple of years later in favor of chartreuse chiffon prom dresses (obviously).

The point is to say that fashion—especially when your choices are a little on the "out there" side, as mine have been from time to time over the years—isn't just about clothing. Pajama pants, ball gowns, or regular old T-shirts and jeans . . . they're not just things that you put on your body in order to not be naked when you go about the day's activities. They're a way of speaking to the world, and they're just one of the many tools that the world uses to figure out who, exactly, you are. What you put on your body can in a very real way express how you see yourself . . . and where you want to go.

Another thing about fashion: It's hugely subjective. As we've seen, one person's "awesome pajama fashion statement" is another person's "runaway teenager attire." And all those differences—those enormous divides in terms of how people interpret fashion and what they believe that a simple piece of fabric can reveal about the wearer—can get you into a spot of trouble from time to time (hopefully not of the "in the back of a police car" variety, but you never know) . . . but really, when it comes down to it, they're great. Because difference breeds experimentation, and experimentation breeds conversation, and from conversation comes change. Evolution.

But there's a weird truth about getting pregnant, and becoming a mom, and that's that it feels, in some ways, like the world's expectations for you shift. You suddenly start feeling like you "should" start being more responsible . . . practical . . . "mom-like." And maybe it's you who starts feeling like minidresses aren't really your thing anymore. Or maybe it's others telling you that it's time to take a turn for the maternally-attired.

Do you know, I once had a reader comment under a fashion post I put up when I was a few months along to alert me to the fact that wearing things like shorts and high heels would be "humiliating" to my future child? Sure, I'm on the Internet, and that puts me in a strange world where very different social/religious/moral spheres collide in ways that they ordinarily wouldn't in "real life," to sometimes dramatic effect, and sure, everyone is entitled to their opinion, but still: I have to disagree. Strongly.

My feeling is that personal appearance is a personal choice, just one of the many exciting decisions that one gets to make for oneself over the course of life. And as for my son? I think I'd rather let him know that it's not for us to judge others based on what makes them happy, and show him that it's cool to be exactly who you are by acting as a handy-dandy, high-heels-and-shorts-wearing Real Live Example.

Even when you're a new mama, you still get to be yourself. And if that means wearing stilettos to the grocery store or bunny slippers 24/7, that is *your decision to make*. Being respectful, being thoughtful, being mindful both of others and of yourself . . . all of those things are important.

But so is being brave.

Being you.

I have years of experience with people telling me that I can't or shouldn't wear one thing or another. And at the end of it all, you know what I say?

Get your glitter eye shadow on if you want to. Just don't also throw on a pair of pajamas in the dead of winter and run around a bus station like a crazy lady. That's just common sense.

A Quick Break with Reality

I have this website called Ramshackle Glam. And on this website I tend to post the odd picture or fifty of myself. And you can call that "fun!" or "crazy vain!" or "overkill!"—because yes, all of those things variously apply—but one thing that this tendency of mine most certainly can be called is "kind of unfortunate when you just gave birth to an entire human being and have promised to shoot and publish a bunch of the aforementioned photos of yourself while wearing actual clothing (as opposed to muumuus) five days later."

Let's talk misguided expectations for a moment.

When I was pregnant, you see, I really for serious did not get it, and by "it" I mean the fact that childbirth is a slightly more strenuous experience than, say, a Pilates class. As an example: About a month before I was due to give birth, I got a call from the producer of a very prominent, very fancy television show asking if I would be interested in coming on as a featured guest. Now, before you get all intimidated by the sheer enormity of my fame and importance and close this book because you can't handle basking in the glory of all this fabulousness for one more second, let me be clear: Offers like this weren't exactly the norm for me. And by "not exactly the norm for me," I mean "had never happened before, ever." My excitement level while on this phone call was hovering somewhere around the hyperventilating/dying/passing out level.

The date of the taping? You guessed it: That very, very special day that I had so carefully marked on my calendar nine months earlier. And my answer when this producer asked whether I was available?

"Oh, sure!"

"But . . . I just wanted to check, because I hear you're pregnant. When are you due?"

"Ah . . . that day, actually."

(Long silence.)

"Oh, but it's no big deal; I mean, what are the chances I'll give birth on the exact date I'm supposed to? If it happens before we tape I'll just pop over afterward! My husband will watch the baby! No worries!"

Did I mention that the segment they wanted me to shoot involved *physically sprinting around New York City on a madcap race to find Manhattan's very best home décor deals*? It did.

I know. I can't explain this break with reality either; I swear I'm not usually this off-the-rails. I was correct in my determination that children rarely go skipping out of your body on the precise day that they're expected to . . . but maybe slightly remiss in my announcement that—no worries!—I would be more than capable of moseying on over to a soundstage for a full-day taping (including madcap sprints!) without even a post-delivery nap, if that's what it took. Fortunately, the producer understood that there was some kind of major hormonal issue happening and that it was interfering with my sanity, and told me very nicely that they'd go ahead and call me in for another segment at some point in the future. They didn't, but I can't say I blame them, because they clearly thought I was out of my mind.

Back to that unfortunate tendency to publish photos of myself on the Internet, and yet another stunning example of my genuine belief that I would be able to windmill myself straight up from that hospital bed and back into my regular routine through sheer force of will. A couple of weeks before I was due to give birth, I signed a contract with a shoe company (the biggest contract of my career up until that point) to style and shoot a series of photographs of myself wearing their products . . . and part of the contract specified that I had to take and publish those photos on certain dates. Dates that ended up being approximately fifty seconds following my arrival home from the hospital with a grouchy newborn and a very nervous husband in tow and a less-than-wonderful sensation taking up residence in 90 percent of my body. Removing my yoga pants and putting on for-real clothing with for-real snaps and buttons over my super-sexy maternity underwear—and then photographing the results—wasn't high on the list of things I was dying to do.

Remember that angry water buffalo I mentioned back in the introduction to this book? Well, putting on high heels made her angrier.

But I was excited about the job, needed the money, and I felt lucky to have the contract, and so guess what? Snaps were snapped, buttons were buttoned, and the photos actually came out pretty well, thanks to a few handy little tricks and go-to pieces. Tricks and go-to pieces that—ba da da!—I am more than thrilled to share with you, my new mama friend.

Postpartum Pulled-Together: Tips and Tricks

It's just a fact of pregnancy: For a few weeks (or, more likely, months), you're going to be dealing with some Baby Leftovers, whether that's a bunch of weight that just won't go away, Breastfeeding-Sized Boobs (we'll talk more about those later, because they deserve their own moment in the sun), loose skin, stretch marks, or some lovely combination of the above. (For me, the hangers-on were The Boobs and The Muffins . . . and not the delicious, chocolate-chip-covered kind of muffins; the "located directly at the precise spot where your waistband makes them most obvious and will not leave no matter what you do" kind.) Not to mention the sleep deprivation, the oceans of zit-inducing hormones coursing through your veins, and the fact that you may or may not be on the receiving end of a seriously enormous—and quite fun, actually—dose of pain medication.

In short: Chances are, this is not the moment you'd choose for a trip down the red carpet. Or a trip to the grocery store.

Before we get going on my favorite what-to-wear tips and must-have pieces for making your new mama self feel like facing the world, let me make this totally clear: *it is okay to feel less than your absolute best for a while.* You just went through something extraordinary and difficult and life-changing and amazing, and it will take time for you to physically feel phenomenal—or like anything even approaching your pre-pregnancy self—again. Carrying and giving birth to a child takes bravery, and it takes strength, and I believe from the bottom of my heart that the very best thing that you can do for yourself in the postpartum period is to chill out a little and take it easy on yourself while your body and mind recover and readjust to their new circumstances. And if what makes you feel best during that readjustment period are enormous pajamas with ducks on them and neon scrunchies, I say go for it.

But sometimes you might *not* want to do that, or might not be able to for whatever reason . . . and that's where I come in.

Now, do I have nutrition/exercise tips for you? I most certainly do not; go ask Dr. Oz or Jillian Michaels or someone who isn't me about that stuff, because I am a Kraft Mac-loving, hot yoga-hating, card-carrying Lazy Person and know exactly nothing about what one should and should not do to whip oneself into shape. What I *do* know about, though, is finding easy ways to feel at least respectably pulled-together when those must-get-dressed-and-face-the-world occasions come around, so let's go!

WHAT YOU'LL NEED

FLOATY, BOHO DRESSES. I'll be honest: I kind of favor the potato-sack look in my day-to-day life generally, but especially when pregnant and right afterward. I know that some people worry about looking like the aforementioned potato in an unstructured piece, but I found that lightweight, relaxed-fit dresses were a great option all the way through my pregnancy and in the weeks and months that followed. Mostly because these kinds of dresses are no-brainers: You can just grab one, throw it on, and go, and you don't have to fuss around wondering whether or not your button will be able to say hey to your buttonhole.

If you're worried about looking too shapeless, no problem: You can always add a skinny belt around your waist or a wider belt slung low across your hips. Another bonus: Boho-style dresses let you feel all ethereal and Earth Mama-y while wafting around the house with your precious, slumbering little angel. (At least for approximately thirty seconds, after which he is guaranteed to excrete something that shatters the illusion.)

WRAP DRESSES. If the bohemian look isn't your thing, try a wrap dress in a comfortable material. I know, it seems like wrap dresses would emphasize your waist in a please-don't-do-that way, but the slight ruching effect that the wrap creates can be very forgiving, and you can adjust the belt to hit you at the part of your torso that you feel is most flattering to your figure (for most people, that's wherever they're smallest).

SCARVES. Scarves are your best friend when it comes to subtly disguising anything from Breastfeeding Boobs to a few extra pounds: The draping creates so much visual interest that it's hard to tell what's fabric and what's figure. They're also a great way to make even the simplest clothing (like a slouchy black T-shirt and a pair of wide-leg black pants, aka my At-Home New Mama Uniform) instantly look like an "outfit."

A PERFECT BLAZER. All right, this is a big one: Throwing on a perfectly tailored, lightweight blazer is the number one way to instantly look like you're capable of existing in Grown-up Land. One caveat: I know you're busy with the whole "new baby at home" thing, but this is not a piece to snag off the Internet; to find the right fit, you'll need to actually try the blazer on in person. It's worth it, though, because once you find your perfect blazer you'll wear it constantly . . . and because you can use your "But honey, Jordan told me I need to buy a blazer!" excuse to also squeeze in a pedicure. Your partner will survive.

- Try pairing a dark blazer with a lighter-colored top to create the visual illusion of a smaller waist.

BELLS AND WHISTLES. You know how Coco Chanel said that before you leave the house, you should look at yourself in the mirror and remove one thing? Well, Coco and I are going to have to agree to disagree, because I am happily enrolled in The School of Pile It On. Of course you'll have to choose your pieces with care (see table, below) but when you're feeling blah, nothing perks you up like a little sparkle.

INSTEAD OF	CHOOSE
Hoops that little fingers can grab	Chunky stud earrings
Long, bulky necklaces with heavy pendants	Collarbone-skimming chains
Bracelets loaded with scratchy gemstones	Slim, elegant bangles
Oversized cocktail rings	Simple mixed-metal stacks

ADORABLE FLATS. Before I had a baby, my shoes fell into two categories: five-inch, vaguely (or, okay, very) stripper-esque heels . . . and flip-flops. In other words, I was either teetering down a street or schlepping down it. When I had my son, though, I quickly realized that simultaneous baby-wrangling and high-heel-wearing posed much too much of a challenge to my already limited balancing capabilities, and decided to start embracing The Flats. Even the most comfortable slip-on shoes can be completely chic: Just go for a classic nude or black (or animal-print) pair with a streamlined shape and minimal embellishment. (Bonus points for toe cleavage; I think it's sexy.)

A RUBBER BAND. Remember that rubber band that you looped through your buttonhole and used to keep your jeans closed early in pregnancy, before you invested in for-real maternity denim or one of those waistband-expanding belt things? Break it out again, because while it's very exciting and fun to get back into the pants you were wearing before you started to show . . . they probably don't fit *quite* yet. Guess what? No one but you has to know. Just finish off your look with a long tank or tee to hide your mini-deception, and let everyone bask in the wonder of your pre-pregnancy-pants-wearing self.

A PHENOMENAL BAG WITH LOTS OF COMPARTMENTS (THE "NON-DIAPER-BAG DIAPER BAG"). When I was pregnant, one indulgence that I knew I wanted to splurge on was a gorgeous diaper bag. Splurge I did, and it was super-cute, and every single time I slung my designer diaper bag over my shoulder I felt like an extremely hot mama. But as it turns out, I could have saved a bunch of cash . . . because I quickly learned that any old bag will do, provided that it's spacious, has a bunch of compartments inside to hold things like pacifiers (which, in my experience, have a tendency to disappear into black holes), and is made of a reasonably easy-to-clean fabric. The one thing I absolutely insist on is that you love it to pieces, because a drop-dead handbag is the single easiest way to instantly spiff up an outfit and make you look like you've got places to go, people to see, babies to change.

SUNGLASSES. When my son was born I became a professional grower of under-eye bags, and I literally do not leave the house without a fantastic pair of oversized sunglasses. Sometimes I wear them at home, too. Because I'm just that tired.

A PIECE OR TWO THAT SPOTLIGHTS YOUR GORGEOUSNESS. Everyone has their "thing" that they love. Great shoulders, beautiful hands, fantastic legs . . . whatever. You've got it. Show it off.

Let's Talk About Those Boobs,
Because They Deserve a Moment to Shine

Every time I visited a lingerie shop during the year or so that I was pregnant and/or breastfeeding, I was struck anew by just how truly out-of-control gigantic my cup size was. You'd think at some point I'd be all, "Well that's just what's happening right now," and move on with my day. But nope. I never got over it.

Which makes sense. I mean, it's kind of hard to "get over" something when it is both making you look like a porn star and feel like Rocky Balboa after a run-in with Apollo Creed.

It was The Boobs, actually, that I found most challenging when it came to pulling together a post-pregnancy wardrobe: I really didn't want to showcase my new additions for everyone on the 6 train to take a gander at . . . but I also had to make sure they were good and ready when they were called into action. Basically, I wanted them to be simultaneously tucked away and completely available. No problem, right?

GO-TO BREAST FEEDING PIECES

The most important thing, of course, is that whatever you're wearing make it easy for you to breast-feed . . . but that doesn't mean that you totally have to sacrifice comfort and style.

TOPS WITH (SOME) BUTTONS. Button-down tops are ideal in theory, but I found it difficult to find button-downs that suited what had become a rather extreme shape. As an alternative, consider tops that button only part-way down (like henleys) made in a comfortable, breathable fabric; they keep you looking chic and streamlined while still making feeding your newborn as easy as pie.

MEMORY RINGS

Some people can always tell which side they last nursed on, but sometimes—like if your baby doesn't eat a whole lot in a given nursing session—it can be hard to remember. Try using a memory ring (a slim gold or silver band that sits just below your first knuckle) to jog your memory: When you've finished a feeding, just transfer it over to the other hand and you'll know where to start next time.

SHIRTS WITH STRETCH. Tops that can easily be pulled down and to the side work well, but take care to choose a style that won't be ruined by a little yanking here and there: Go for a cotton blend with some stretch to it, or even a wrap top (which can also be adjusted as your post-baby body changes, making it a good investment). Cowl-neck tops are also a good pick, because the extra fabric allows you to shift the neckline around as needed.

NURSING TANKS. If you're wearing a top that you'll need to pull up from the waistline, you might want to layer a nursing tank (or just a regular lightweight tank top) underneath so that you don't feel too exposed.

PRETTY SCARVES. Burp cloths can always be used for extra concealment, but beautiful, lightweight scarves can double as cover-ups in a pinch. And if you feel like your brand-new cup size is making your regular wardrobe a little too risqué for your taste, you can just loop the scarf around your neck for extra coverage once you're done nursing.

JUST SAY NO TO SILK. Put down the dry-clean-only pieces for the time being. It's not worth it.

To clarify: In my opinion, all these tips apply to in-public appearances only. If putting on a cute top and a floral scarf while you're just hanging around the house happens to make you feel great, do it up . . . but if not, just go ahead and wear whatever makes life easiest, even if what makes life easiest is "nothing." Hey, it's your house; you'll be naked if you want to.

Speaking of Naked . . .

You know that saying, "She'd lose her head if it wasn't screwed onto her body"? (Or something like that.)

Well, that's me.

As an example: These days it would not be out of the realm of possibility for me to leave the house without pants on.

The thing about breastfeeding is that it's a hell of a lot easier if you stay in a state of partial disrobement at all times. And because this style of dressing has started to feel normal, I've had to remind myself on occasion that this is not an appropriate state in which to greet the FedEx guy or assorted other visitors. Yesterday I took the baby over to the doctor's office, and halfway there I felt a chill in a place where a chill should not be, and had to frantically check to make sure that I was in fact wearing leggings, and hadn't accidentally put on tights and forgotten to add the requisite something-to-go-over-them. As it turned out, I was happily covered up—just not wearing enough layers—but I am constantly doing things like leaving the house to walk the dogs wearing a T-shirt, jeans, and flip-flops. In January.

And you know what? A couple of times I've just said "F it" and continued on my dog-walking way. Because once you've wrestled a baby in a bear suit, a panicking lhasa apso, and a near-comatose shih tzu down four flights of stairs, hypothermia seems like a better option than prolonging the experience for one more second than absolutely necessary.

What's obviously going on here is that I'm so preoccupied with making sure that the baby has the gazillion things he needs in order to leave our little nest happily and safely that I'm completely forgetting to attend to my own attire. Whatever goes on my body is usually the fastest and easiest thing to put on when I'm already fifteen minutes late. (Because despite the fact that I have historically prided myself on being to-the-letter on-time, I am now always fifteen minutes late.) Just saying: If you see me walking down the street, and I'm not wearing pants . . . maybe give me a heads-up?

Starting from Scratch:
New Life, New Wardrobe

A few months after I started writing Ramshackle Glam, I put up my very first "personal style" post. It was a couple of days before New Year's Eve, and while my actual New Year's agenda involved a very glamorous lineup of my husband's pajama pants, cheap champagne, and a zombie movie or two, it occurred to me that it would be fun to write about what I would have worn had I actually made plans involving . . . I don't know, a ballroom or something. And to illustrate this mini-fantasy with photos.

So I put on a floor-length yellow silk gown that I'd bought at a sample sale a few months earlier (forgetting that my life never, ever involves occasions to which one might conceivably wear a floor-length yellow silk gown), topped it with a faux fur vest (because why not?) . . . and then finished the whole thing off with a pair of navy rain boots, because it was snowing outside and that was just the way it was.

Then I lugged my camera and tripod up to my roof (because it had great light), and ran around in the snow taking photos of the whole deal. And then I put those photos on the Internet.

Obviously.

Now, I'm aware that for much of the population doing something like this is considered "weird" . . . but honestly: In retrospect, you know what I think the weirdest part was?

The fact that my decision to shoot my very first style post was preceded by this exact thought: "Hmm . . . I wonder what I should do this afternoon."

Nowadays, that is not a question that enters my mind. Everrr.

The number of things that I have to do in the next *minute* of my life hovers somewhere around 3,453, and I am always (always, always) aware of every. single. one of them.

I mean that.

I am aware of the things that I have to do the moment my eyes pop open in the morning (and I make sure that my husband becomes aware of them at this point in time, too; he loves this). I am aware of the things that I have to do while I am physically doing them. I am aware of them while watching terrible reality TV during "me time" (which is not really "me time" but rather "worry about all the things I'm not doing while pretending to relax" time) before bed, and I am aware of them at 3:00 a.m., when my sleep cycle lightens for a moment and I am instantly startled into wakefulness by the sheer volume of Musts that are awaiting the rise of the sun.

And chances are you feel the same way, because babies have this little habit of sucking up minutes like tiny, turbocharged Dyson vacuums.

In short: I no longer have time to put on gowns and run around in the snow. Or eat a meal while sitting down.

But guess what? Still gotta get dressed! Mostly because while nudity can certainly be fun, it's not really an option in the suburbs (or at least not in my suburb) . . . and because I like clothing. I *like* feeling at least semi-chic; and like I could run into a friend on the street and not want to hide behind a tree.

But when my son was born and my life changed, my approach to pulling together my wardrobe changed, too: I had to figure out ways to look like an approximation of myself while also making sure that the pajamas-to-actual-clothing transformation took no more than three minutes, tops. There is no "trying on a bunch of cute shirts to see which one looks best"; there is just "put on shirt now."

So I whittled my wardrobe down using a very basic formula, and it's a formula that I use *every single day*. And every single day it gets me out of the house ready for whatever the day may bring. . . .

As long as the day doesn't involve ballrooms. Because that floor-length yellow silk gown went in the Give-Away Pile long ago, my friend.

MY EASY NEW-MOM SOLUTION

In the months since my son arrived, the number of items in my closet that I actually *wear* has shrunk enormously. I reach for the same pieces (my favorite pair of skinny jeans, my favorite gray tee, my favorite brown boots) over and over and over . . . because while I still like to have fun with fashion, of course, the fact is that when life gets extra busy, there's something to be said for knowing what works for you, and for being able to look at least somewhat pulled-together virtually on autopilot.

Sometimes when your life undergoes a dramatic shift your wardrobe has to shift right along with it. Maybe you just feel more comfortable hitting up the playground wearing jeans rather than the skirts you used to favor. Maybe you find that nowadays fitted tops are more your vibe than flowy ones. Or maybe you need to switch out the heels for a cute pair of flats because you're just carrying so many damn *things* all the time (on an average day, I carry around the following: one twenty-five-pound toddler; one diaper bag with a missing strap; two dogs who thrive on defiance, hate their leashes, and think that the hill over there looks like a much better place to be; three to five grocery bags; about twenty toy cars, each one of which must be accessible *at all times*; and about ten thousand Cheerios, sometimes in a snack cup and sometimes in my hair.)

But wait! I'm not saying that you have to all of a sudden abandon your beloved minidresses for a Mom Costume consisting of flex-sole sneakers and reindeer sweatshirts. You still get to look like you . . . just a version of you that makes a little more sense in your new life.

All you have to do: Figure out what kind of silhouette you feel best in, make sure that you own a few key mix-and-match pieces, and then integrate eye-catching (but not necessarily expensive) extras.

SILHOUETTE + SPICE = SIMPLE STYLE

STEP 1. FIND YOUR SILHOUETTE. First, let's find the shape that you feel best in. Try this: Pretend you're meeting up with a friend who you haven't seen in a long time; someone you want to look really great for. In a perfect world, what would you wear? A pretty sundress? A fitted tee and jeans? A pencil skirt and blouse? For me, the answer to this question is "a loose, light-weight top and skinny jeans" . . . but whatever your own answer is, that's your "happy place" silhouette, and the one that you should build your wardrobe around.

STEP 2. ADD SPICE. Even when you're starting with basic items, the addition of one or two truly phenomenal accessories can transform what you're wearing from "clothing" into a for-real "outfit." The best part: There's no need to spend a fortune on your accessories; use them to add color, texture, and interest to your look, and then swap them out with the seasons, as trends change, or just because you feel like it.

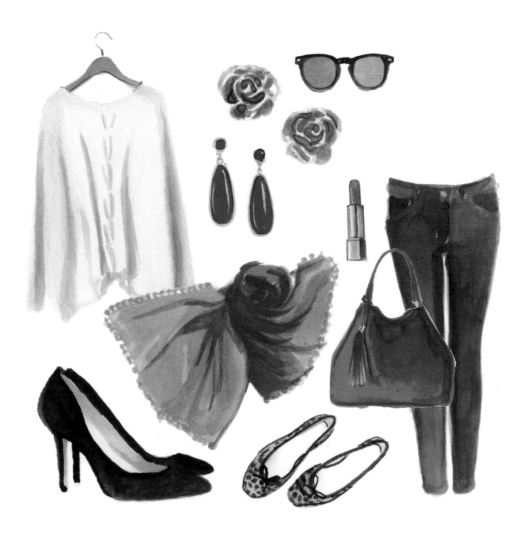

If you choose the right extras, you can end up with a practically infinite number of combinations that can work for everything from errands to dinner with friends to just hanging out around the house. And because you're starting out with a shape you love, you know that you'll feel great in every single one.

BUILDING A WARDROBE FROM SCRATCH

* For your key pieces, shoot for the middle of the road, price-wise: You want quality basics that will hold their shape, but there's no need to spend a fortune.

* If you find a piece that you truly adore, don't be afraid to pick it up in a couple of different colors; on the rare occasion that I find a T-shirt that fits exactly how I like T-shirts to fit, I always buy at least three .

* You'll save a ton of time getting ready in the morning if you toss or store everything that doesn't fit well, that's seen better days, or that you honestly just never really want to wear for whatever reason—the goal is to be able to just reach into your closet, grab whatever you spot first, and be good to go.

* Buy a gorgeous pair of sunglasses (knock-offs work just fine). Nothing will make you feel more "done" in five seconds flat, even on mornings when your little one gets you up extra early.

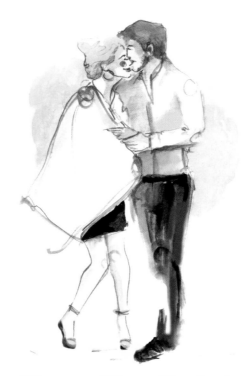

I Never Want to Wear Heels Again
(Date Night)

I fall a lot.

Not in a cute, "oh, look, she's so goofy and just like Zooey Deschanel" way . . . in a fairly cataclysmic way that frequently requires the intervention of one or more total strangers.

And yet, because I am nothing if not stubborn, for years and years I wore heels like they were glued to my feet. Everywhere. In college, my boyfriend used to say that he knew I had entered the dining hall before he even saw me because he heard me clomping over to get my tray. I wore heels shopping (for groceries). I wore them to breakfast. I even wore them on things like cobblestone streets, which are difficult for normal, marginally coordinated human beings to walk on.

I remember once, when I was twenty-two, visiting some adorable little town in Southern California with my mom and my aunt Trudy, and deciding that a day trip with my relatives presented the perfect opportunity to dress like I was going to the *clurrrb* in a flippy little dress and enormous lace-up wedges. When I say that I "fell" that day, I mean that I spent more time during that trip on the ground than on my feet. For real: I bit it approximately every two to three steps, to the point where my poor aunt was practically in tears because she was so worried that I was going to break something important, like my face.

When I got pregnant, I continued to wear my five-inch heels all the way through to the end. I know, I just said I can barely walk when my center of gravity is in its normal state rather than thrown off by an entire human being glued to my midsection, but I wore flats while in transit and just changed into my heels whenever I arrived at my destination (you've honestly never seen "glamorous" until you've seen a seven-months-pregnant lady clinging to a wall outside a restaurant while struggling to jam a pair of stilettos onto her swollen feet).

Once that baby arrived?

DONE.

I mean, it's not like I tossed my platform collection straight out the window and down onto Second Avenue . . . but I am no longer interested in putting anything on my feet that doesn't feel good. I still wear heels, sure, but I will not wear heels that hurt. It's just not going to happen.

And most days, honestly? It's all flats, all the time.

Why the newfound focus on Foot Coziness? Three reasons:

1. When our son was born, we lived in a fourth-floor walk-up apartment in a building that did not permit me to leave the stroller in the lobby downstairs, thereby forcing me to make, at minimum, a thrice-daily trek up and down carrying the following:
   • One baby;

- One diaper bag containing approximately six times the number of things I actually needed to take with me on a three-minute walk to the corner store;
- Assorted shopping bags and Red Bull containers;
- Two dogs that were both extremely tired of living in thirty square feet of space, thanks to the moving boxes filling our entire apartment, and also more than a little ticked off at having been downgraded from Our Beloved Babies to Those Things That Wake Up Our Child When They Bark (Which Is All The Time); and
- One stroller that weighed eighteen pounds on the way down, but magically inflated to twice that size on the way up.

2. The act of walking in heels for more than three blocks has, on occasion, begun to generate crippling, collapse-on-the-ground-style pain-spasms in my feet. Why? I don't know, but I suspect it has something to do with aging and associated bodily disrepair, so let's not dwell.

3. Even on Date Nights . . . I just don't care. Or rather, I care less about looking like a beauty queen than I care about the sense of *freedom*—both emotional and physical—that makes my rare evenings out with my husband so special.

Here's the thing: once your family expands, it's easy to forget what it felt like when it was Just Two (*see* page 147: "Oh Right . . . I'm Married"). And while Date Nights are important because they let you go out, have fun, get a little crazy, do whatever it is you used to do during that courtship phase, what's even *more* important to recapture, if just for a night, is that sense of lightness. Abandon, even.

Along with the wonders of parenthood come responsibilities and obligations beyond anything you—or at least I—have ever experienced before . . . so when I get the chance to take a couple of hours off of my Must List to grab some margaritas with Kendrick, the last thing I want is to feel tied down by a pair of stilettos I can barely walk in. Or by a too-tight dress. Or by anything that is uncomfortable in any way at all; I want the focus to be on *us*, not me.

I want to be able to skip from restaurant to car if skipping is what I feel like doing. And I don't want my heels to stop me.

WHAT TO WEAR: DATE NIGHT

- I'm a firm believer in The Power of Leopard; if you use animal prints sparingly (one item of clothing or accessory per outfit), you can think of them virtually as neutrals. Except they're animal prints. Which is much more fun.

- A perfect pair of pointy-toed nude or black flats or low heels is a wardrobe staple; nothing will make you feel more polished in seconds.

> When it comes to footwear it's all about comfort, so skip online shopping in favor of actually trying the shoes on in the store. This way, you can make sure they'll be able to come with you wherever you want to go.

* The right T-shirt can be totally Date Night–appropriate if you go for a lightweight fabric that moves with your body and a great neckline that draws focus to your face. I especially love slightly-off-the-shoulder styles paired with brightly colored bras with beautiful, show-off-able straps.

* If you want to go for a dress, try a simple, comfortable shape in an unexpected, saturated color.

* Instantly upgrade your LBD with the addition of a couple of statement-making accessories like a cuff bracelet, a sparkly purse that doubles as jewelry, or collarbone-grazing earrings.

* If you're going straight from day to night without much time to fancy up your look, try easy upgrades to add color, sparkle, and a touch of glam.

With My Grown-Up Costume On

When I was in my mid-twenties and working as an actress in Los Angeles, my specialty was playing drug-addicted prostitutes. I'm serious: I could do "distraught and speedy" like nobody's business. There was a period, however, around the time I turned twenty-four, when a rash of law-type shows flooded the networks and suddenly all anyone wanted me to audition for was "bright-eyed newbie attorney who becomes disillusioned by the hard, hard realities of her job." Slightly less fun, perhaps, but hey, work is work.

Unfortunately, this type of work required that I own a suit, and my L.A. closet was mostly filled with bikinis.

So off to Banana Republic I went. I ended up returning home with a simple black blazer and pencil skirt set that may not have actually gotten me any acting jobs, but that certainly made me look slightly less out-of-place while sitting in all those waiting rooms and staring at my scripts. That suit is still hanging in my closet nearly a decade later, and while it's still in good shape and still one of the more pulled-together-looking things I own, I've barely put it on in the years since I left California (and the acting industry). Not even for events for which one might imagine a suit would be required; even if business attire is on the menu, I'd almost always rather look slightly (even inappropriately) underdressed than put on something that makes me so frankly uncomfortable.

The thing is, whenever I wear something like a suit—or any item of clothing, honestly, that says "completely responsible and fully integrated member of society"—I feel like I'm playing dress-up. While I enjoy tiptoeing around on the periphery of all different types of looks, something about the idea of dressing "like a grown-up" (by which I mean polished, sophisticated, a little conservative) often escapes me, and makes me feel I've tried on someone else's skin that doesn't fit quite right. Putting on a suit may make me "look" more like someone able to take care of business, but it makes me feel like hiding.

I do like this look in theory, though, so my discomfort with the tailored side of the spectrum never made a ton of sense to me . . . until I realized that—of course—it's not about clothing at all. (It never actually is.)

Like so many great breakthroughs in life, this one occurred while watching a Will Smith movie (*I Am Legend*; don't judge). There's a scene where Will is carrying his onscreen daughter toward a helicopter, and he's wearing a gorgeous suit and the wind is dramatically flapping the hem of his jacket around, and he just looks so . . . capable. I mean, he was *striding* toward that helicopter. Purposefully. I don't think I've ever strode with that much purpose in my life.

Now, granted (and as my husband, who is reading over my shoulder, just very graciously reminded me): I will never be mistaken for Will Smith, both because of the obvious and because there are few people on the planet who convey a sense of competence quite so well. He'd look exactly like the kind of guy who gets things done whether he was wearing a suit, a ripped T-shirt, or nothing at all.

So that's settled: I will never, ever look as on top of things as Will Smith does. And that's fine, but still: I have to wonder what it is about those style trappings that we traditionally associate with adulthood—a sharply tailored blazer; trouser pants cuffed just-so; a crisp black skirt suit—that make me feel so . . . honestly?

Inadequate.

The thing is that these past couple of years—the years since the birth of our son— have made me think very hard about what it means to be an adult, to be responsible, to keep all those balls in the air: the mortgages, the 529 plans, the retirement accounts, the laundry, the dishes, the job, the relationship, the family, the life. Every second of every day, I'm trying to hold all of these countless must-dos in check, keep them organized and structured and safe . . . and yet so often it feels like all I'm doing is trying to look the part when inside is another person entirely: a little kid who's just worried about getting all of her chores done in time to watch one cartoon before bed.

It constantly blows my mind, the realization that those parents who seemed like they had it all under control—our parents—were just . . . us. They were just people—grown-ups (according to all visible markers, anyway)—who were trying to get through the day without screwing up too badly, and who were maybe feeling like children trying on their daddy's suits as well.

So maybe I don't love wearing "grown-up clothing" because it makes me feel like I'm faking it, and like my costume is fooling exactly no one.

Except.

Sometimes, in the morning, my son will open his eyes and cry: wanting a waffle, wanting orange juice, wanting to be picked up/put down/put in his seat/taken outside. Just *wanting*. And I couldn't figure out was going on with him, until finally I realized: My husband takes a minute to get moving in the morning, too. I'm the kind of person who's checking my emails from bed before I've even turned on the light, but he likes to relax in the minutes after he wakes up, be with himself, not just get up and go go go. And if my husband is like this . . . perhaps, I thought, so is my child. And so I decided to try slowing things down. Rather than popping my son straight into his jeans and rushing him down to the breakfast table, I've started lifting him quietly from the crib and carrying him downstairs, still in his PJs. I leave the lights off and we take a pause, just lie together under a blanket and watch the light flicker in the space heater. Drink some juice. Maybe close our eyes for just a second longer if we need to.

One morning, he seemed to want something extra, and so I picked him up and held him, singing "Ol' 55" into the crook of his neck while we danced around the darkened room.

And I caught sight of myself in the reflection on the TV.

I didn't look like a pulled-together adult; I looked like an exhausted girl in wrinkly pajamas who badly needed to find a hairbrush. But I also looked like a parent who was rocking her baby because that's what he needed. I looked like me: like a daughter and a mother and a child and a woman all at the same time.

Saddle Shoes and Turning Tides

When I was in fifth grade, I attended a private school on New York City's Upper West Side that required its students to wear uniforms: The boys wore slacks and collared shirts, and the girls wore little belted pale-blue jumpers. The popular girls in my class wore the jumpers oversized and beltless, layering them over white or navy turtlenecks that were bunched at the neck (never rolled). My mom said that they looked "messy" and packed me off to school in button-down blouses with enormous, frilly collars, my belt tied on exactly where it was supposed to go.

I was not cool, not even a little bit.

I took a sort of pride in my non-coolness; sometimes it even felt like a thing that I had chosen rather than a thing that just was. One week, all the girls decided to wear their scrunchies around their ankles, but I elected to keep my scrunchie in my hair where it belonged, mostly because the concept of putting it on my foot struck me as both pointless and confusing. My choice to buck that particular trend made me feel pretty good, actually . . . in a small way it felt like a sign that I was doing my own thing, and that "my own thing" might be a kind of awesome thing to do.

Then, in the spring of that year, everyone (by which I mean Sarah and Nell and Katie and the other girls I wanted very badly to be just like) started wearing saddle shoes. I *loved* them. I wanted a pair of my own. But I felt silly about the fact that I wanted them; it seemed embarrassing to even desire an item that was so clearly what the popular kids were into. I worried that it would seem like I was wearing them just to fit in, or that "fitting in" was actually what I did want.

And maybe it was.

But either way: I really liked those shoes.

A month or so went by, and I finally caved: I went to my mother and asked for a pair. She said no at first—they were way too expensive—but a bit more begging finally did her in. I wore my saddle shoes to school the very next Monday, on the exact day that every single other girl in school decided that saddle shoes were not only no longer "in" . . . they were supremely dorky and would only be worn by total nerds.

I wish I could say that I wore them anyway, but I didn't. My mom was mad, but the saddle shoes stayed in my closet all summer long, and by the next fall they were too small and that was that.

It's funny, but despite the fact that I really do deep-down believe that you should wear what you want to wear and to hell with what anyone has to say about it . . . I still think of those saddle shoes from time to time, when some crazy trend or another arises: tangerine lipstick, chalk-dyed hair, peplum. Sometimes I want to try that trend out myself just because it seems like it'd be fun, or because I actually do like it despite the fact that it might make me look a little odd, but a tiny voice from way, way back pipes up in my head, worrying about things like turning tides and laughing girls.

When I became a mom, my style changed a lot. The essence of it—the slouchiness, the off-the-shoulder cuts, the obsession with denim shorts and leopard-print—

remained the same, but some things—like, say, leather pants that I could barely bend over in—simply didn't accommodate the demands of my new life. My mornings grew too busy to allow me to play around with my closet the way I used to. And sometimes, I admit, I've wondered if a little of the fun has drained away.

In the spring of 2013, wedge sneakers started popping up in celebrity magazines. I thought they were the most hideous things I'd ever seen, and immediately slotted them into the "not me, never never never" box.

And then I saw them again. And again.

And suddenly I really, really liked them.

I felt a little ridiculous about it for a moment—liking something that was so obviously a trend, and that would so clearly be a Fashion Moment to roll one's eyes over in a few years—if not a few months—but then I realized:

I don't care.

Yeah, they're funny-looking, but they're also comfortable, and they make me happy when I put them on. So I picked up a pair of wedge sneakers of my very own, and spent a blissful Saturday chasing my son all over Manhattan's American Museum of Natural History in them. I emerged with nary a blister . . . and feeling fabulous, if I have to tell the truth.

I'm not in fifth grade anymore. I don't have to wear a belt with my dress if I don't feel like it, and if I want to wear the shoes that everyone else is wearing?

That's exactly what I'm going to do.

Because fashion is not about rules and must-nots and who-thinks-what-about-who. When it comes down to it, fashion is really just dressing up, and it should be fun. Wild. Even ridiculous, sometimes.

So I'm going to go ahead and wear my wedge sneakers whenever I feel like it, thanks very much.

Later?

Who knows. Either way: it's my call.

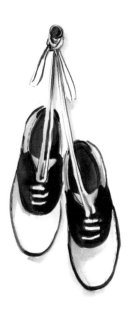

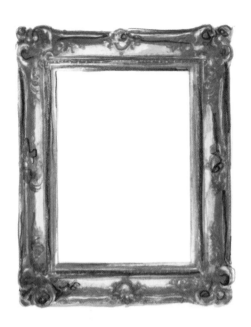

Beauty

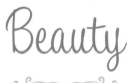

(Your Hair Is Awesome, and That's a Good Start)

Where All the Almosts Lie

For nearly two decades now, I have made it my business to come face-to-face with my own image daily, whether by choice or by chance or by vanity or by some combination of the three. In my present career, I spend a good deal of time thinking about—and then standing in front of cameras and talking about—things like makeup tips; fashion and décor ideas; little ways to add beauty to your day that hopefully make you feel good. Happy. But I know that it's not always that simple—the question of when and how and why one feels beautiful, and what all that has to do with genuine happiness—because it wasn't always that simple for me.

Years ago, in my mid-twenties, I thought much too much about what I looked like and what my ability to achieve a very specific idea I had of beauty might mean for my career (and, by extension, my life . . . because at that point neither was going particularly well, and yet the two seemed neatly tied up in each other). Nearly everything that I thought about beauty at the time—what it was, how I might go about transforming myself, what that transformation might accomplish—was inaccurate, as it turned out, but still: These ideas filled up my mind, leaving very little room for anything else. I spent my days searching for ways to cover myself up, show people something different than what *was*, and rushing through the hours of daylight so that I could start looking for happiness somewhere out there in the night, where the music was playing loudly enough that I wouldn't have to listen to anything else at all.

Right after I graduated from college, I moved out to Los Angeles to "work" as an actress, which mostly just meant wandering around various Coffee Bean & Tea Leafs hoping that my phone would ring, and that it would be my agent calling to tell me that I'd booked that guest spot on *Lost*. Months went by, the days blending together, pockmarked by slow walks to buy groceries or to pick up dry cleaning, drives down the block to take the car through the car wash even though it didn't really need it. I grew sad for reasons that I understood and for reasons that would take me years to unwrap, and the sadness was so big that it pushed other things—most things, really—out of the way. It felt like I was wandering through an endless maze of "almosts": Every day, I made turns that led me to places where I almost got the job, almost had the career, almost changed my life . . . but usually those turns just ended up taking me right on back to the beginning again.

Each morning when I opened my eyes, I started over.

I was so sad, and yet felt *so close*, just a single breath away from what I imagined happiness might be like. I thought maybe, maybe, it might be just one small, simple thing that would make the difference between the life I had and the life I wanted.

It was too scary to imagine that the thing making the difference might be talent, or luck, or even just a simple game of numbers that came down to the fact that the town in which I was living and trying to work was filled with hundreds—thousands—of girls just like me. Worst of all, it might not have had anything to do with my career at all; it might have been something far bigger, far more frightening, far more difficult to put a finger on. It might have been *me*, might have been that broken record in my head saying "can't can't can't."

It was easier to think that maybe that thing keeping me from the life I hoped was waiting for me—the life I thought I "deserved," for no particularly good reason other than that in my head *of course* I deserved it, of course I did—was something as small as hair that was just a shade blonder, a waist that was just a hint narrower: Change that one tiny thing, I thought, and there I'd be. I convinced myself that perhaps if I felt beautiful—*was* beautiful—everything would turn out just as I hoped, and so I glossed my lips, bronzed my skin, and covered up my eyes as best as I could, and then smiled like I meant it.

In the Land of Time

I spent the summer of the year I turned twenty-two living in a movie star's house in Malibu. My boyfriend's best friend had flown off to Italy to marry a famous actress, and so my boyfriend and I packed up his new puppy and moved into the actress's seaside mansion to spend a couple of months looking after her home and her pets. It sounds like a terrible hardship, I know: The property was on a cliff overlooking the ocean, and every morning we drank our coffee sitting by the pool, watching dolphins and whales surfacing just offshore.

But the reality of it wasn't nearly as idyllic as it sounds. The actress's dogs (all twenty of them) very obviously wanted to kill me, my relationship was unraveling more and more every week, and I spent most days pacing around the guest house while my boyfriend did whatever he did in the upstairs office of the main house. If someone came to visit, they probably weren't there to see me; I was still relatively new to L.A., and hadn't made many friends.

We had cell phones, but they didn't work way out by the ocean, so one day we strung soda cans from window to window in case we wanted to chat without running back and forth between houses.

We never used them.

I don't know how to explain how I felt in those days better than this: I could barely see straight through the crushing loneliness, through the fact that I couldn't find a single thing in my mind or in my future that I thought would make me happy . . . but still, I tried—hard—to find beauty where I could. Even in moments when I thought I might be sadder than I'd ever been before, I was still aware that I was standing on a windswept beach with lighthouses blinking way off in the dark water.

I had this vision, that summer, of what the future might be like if I wished very, very hard: I'd be a glamorous actress married to a successful screenwriter, and we'd live in a beautiful waterfront home with our sweet pets and sandy-footed children. Every night we'd cook steaks and asparagus on our barbecue, and then I'd wrap myself in layers of white gauze and pad barefoot to our big wooden bed before falling asleep to the sound of crashing waves. The only thing was, I couldn't see any faces in that vision: It was all just sand and water and barking dogs and white cotton tangled up in clean sheets.

Because even though if you squinted your eyes very hard my life at that moment didn't look all that different from the one I imagined for myself, what I really was, was an unhappy girl with an angry boyfriend and a dog who didn't really even belong to me, living in an uncomfortable place where everything was damp and nothing was ours, and no desire to cook anything at all.

So I sat alone in our movie star–sized Malibu bedroom and put my hair up, then put it down, waiting for the phone call that I thought would change it all. I thought a lot about my face, and whether it was enough in a world where it seemed like faces were everything, and decided that it probably wasn't. I rearranged the pillows on the bed, moved them back to where they had been before. I fixed my hair again.

And I drove: Back and forth, up and down along the coast. Sometimes I stopped for frozen yogurt and window-shopping. Sometimes I just kept on driving, waiting for the light to change.

Hairy Legs, Schmary Legs

When I was twelve years old, a director who lived in my apartment building asked me to audition for a commercial. That audition led to me signing with an agent and appearing on things like Frosted Flakes commercials and *Law & Order* episodes. I modeled for Jordache Jeans, and once was carried down a runway by two men while wearing a wedding dress and holding a whip. I played Hugh Hefner's daughter in a biopic and got mildly hit on by the actor playing my dad. I read a lot of books while sitting in trailers and waiting for my turn.

Being a teenage actress was alternately very exciting and kind of embarrassing, and ended up being my post-college career for a few years, until I realized that I kind of hate acting and am actually not particularly good at it.

When I was twelve, however, becoming a professional actress did many important things for my life, including allow me to purchase my daily Tasti D-Lite with my very own money, meet Benjamin Bratt, and occasionally miss school in order to do stuff like hang out on a beach eating seafood (Red Lobster commercial) or sit on the hood of a pickup truck looking wistful (music video). But the most important thing that my job did for my twelve-year-old self? Easy—it convinced my mother to buy me two things: a beeper (pink, sparkly, *themostamazingthingever*) and a black Filofax with a snap cover that made me feel enormously grown-up and important, and that was supposed to help me keep track of my auditions.

What it did instead was kick-start a long and prolific career in obsessive list-making.

Despite the fact that I am the opposite of a hoarder and really prefer to throw out or give away absolutely everything that isn't hugely or immediately useful, I still have that Filofax tucked away in a keepsakes box in my attic, because the extensiveness with which I documented every single thing on my teenage to-do list transformed it into a type of diary. I mean, seriously, there were *illustrations* in that thing. Charts.

I'm still big on lists to this day. I keep notes in my phone tracking everything from Christmas gift ideas to frequent flier numbers to recipes I'd like to try. My daily to-dos are written out each morning in little lined booklets stacked next to my computer, and anytime an errand (no matter how menial) pops into my mind it goes straight into my phone's calendar without even a second of reflection. If all that documenting and duplicating sounds excessive, let me assure you: It may make me a little crazy . . . but it also makes me eminently on top of my shit. Which is *awesome*.

The positive side effect of all this list-keeping and note-taking is that I don't have to actually remember anything, ever.

The negative side effect? Same thing.

If it's not written down in my iPhone, it's not going to happen. Simple as that.

Guess what hasn't made the list lately? Any activity whatsoever involving a razor and shaving cream.

You know, right before I went into the hospital to have my son I remember being extra caught up in the idea of making sure that everything was just-so, and my lists started jumping the shark straight from "detailed" into "insane." Even I look at my lists from that time period (they're still saved and backed-up; see: obsessive) and think, "Jesus, lady. You're giving birth to a child, not trying to assemble an Ikea Baby from scratch without an instruction manual. People have done it before. Go drink some tea."

On the prebirth lists that I made were smart things, like reminders to myself not to forget to bring the car seat to the hospital or to pick up stamps so that I could send out thank-you cards for the registry gifts before an infant arrived to occupy my thank-you card-writing hand. And also things like a fully itemized list of every single item of clothing I should wear on the five-minute journey from our apartment to the hospital, because making my grand entrance at the maternity ward garbed in that exact shirt with my nails painted that exact shade of pink seemed very, very important. Because I'm ridiculous.

Supporting evidence for that assertion: In addition to planning out an outfit that (I would soon learn) would be removed from my person mere seconds after my arrival at the hospital, I also calendared shaving appointments with myself every two days leading up to my due date. You know, so as not to stun my doctor with the realization that sometimes women grow hair on their legs.

Which brings me to my point, and my point is this: When I say to you that I can't remember the last time I shaved my legs, I mean it. I can't. But I just checked, and they're actually reasonably non-wooly, which means that some kind of autopilot appears to have kicked in that enables me to occasionally pick up a razor and haphazardly apply it to my legs without ever realizing that such a thing is taking place. And that's nice, I suppose.

It's not that I don't care; I do. And it's not that I'm awesomely wise and non-vain now; I'm not, and I totally still am. It's just that I used to be the kind of person who shaved just because a couple of days had gone by and it was probably time—the kind of person who really, honestly never left the house without at least something on her face (definitely a little powder, maybe a little mascara). And now it's not unusual for five o'clock to roll around without me ever even having glanced in the mirror. Even when I do want to put on some makeup and fix my hair, there's no way that I'm dedicating more than five minutes to the task, because that's five minutes that could really be spent doing more important things. Like drinking coffee. Or eating something that requires a fork.

I'll tell you what though: In my pre-baby life, when I did things like play around with different shades of eye shadow on a Saturday evening just because hey, why not? . . . I would've thought that this would have bothered me, at least a little.

But it doesn't.

Because not only have I realized that—ba da dum!—my self-worth isn't actually tied to my ability to apply liquid eyeliner before a trip to CVS . . . I've also discovered that looking "good" or "pulled-together" or "like a human being who has slept, ever" isn't about half an hour spent sitting in front of the mirror. It's simple, actually.

(Okay, a few tricks are involved. But they're easy ones, I swear!)

Hair Today, Gone Tomorrow

Around the five-month mark in my pregnancy, I began to notice that my hair was the kind of phenomenal reserved for supermodels and women who wear Ralph Lauren. I'd assumed the "your hair doesn't fall out when you're pregnant" thing was an old wives' tale, but nope. Never in my life has my hair been as spectacular as it was during the eight or so months surrounding the birth of my child.

You know how people who have, say, really amazing skin are all "Oh, this old thing?" about it? They're just so used to hearing how *amaaaaazing* their skin is from every single person in the world that by the time you get around to delivering your compliment they sort of give that bored half-smile that extremely attractive celebrities give when they get complimented on anything, ever? Well, by the time my son was born, that was how I was acting about my hair: as if for my entire life it hadn't been a half-wavy, half-straight semi-conundrum, and had always been lovely and horse mane-y and full and shiny. *Obviously.*

And then I stopped breast-feeding.

And it all fell out.

Like, immediately. All of it.

Now, they (by which I mean my mom and a pregnancy book I read) warn you that this is going to happen as a result of the abrupt drop in your estrogen levels, but I had decided I was a Magical Pregnancy Hair Unicorn who had skipped straight from Blessed with Temporary Hair-Benefiting Hormones That Bless Everyone Who Is Pregnant to Straight-Up Blessed, 'Cause I'm Lucky Like That, and was completely unprepared for the handfuls—I'm serious: *handfuls*—of hair that came out of my head every single time I took a shower. I started saving these handfuls to show to my husband, because I needed someone else to be as freaked out as I was. I even tried a little Schopenhauer-style manipulation on my scalp, willing it to hold on to those absconding follicles for dear life.

Needless to say, visualization exercises are no match for biology: By the time my son hit six months old, every single one of those luscious extra strands had hit the road. Then, over the course of the next few months, I discovered an added bonus: regrowth that created a stunning halo of two-inch-long hairs that swam out from my scalp in every direction, making it appear as if I had stuck my fingers into an electric socket every time I pulled my hair into a ponytail.

Do I miss my Pregnancy Unicorn hair? I do. It was really pretty. But as with all the other dramas that come along with new motherhood, the mini-disasters that happen on your scalp are totally manageable.

You just need a few tools at the ready, that's all.

How-To: HANDLE THAT HAIR LOSS

First of all, know that while your hair may feel thinner than usual now, it'll return to its normal state soon (usually around the one-year mark). In the meantime, try playing around with products and styling techniques that create the illusion of thickness.

- Scrunching a dollop of mousse into damp hair before blow-drying

- Switching your part to the other side

- Cutting your hair above your shoulders or adding layers

- Adding highlights: the chemical process roughs up hair strands, and the visual contrast between the colors adds depth

How-To: HANDLE THE BABY HAIR HALO

After all that hair falls out, it's going to grow back in, which is great . . . but if you're anything like me, that stage can also be a touch awkward. If you notice a little corona of short hairs around your head every time you pull your hair into an elastic, just mist a brush with hairspray and lightly pass it over the spots that could use a little extra taming. If the hairs are extra-tiny, you can even use a natural-bristle toothbrush (not the one you brush your teeth with, obviously) to smooth them down.

Stop the Madness: An Ounce of Prevention

A couple of years after I graduated from college and moved to L.A. my boyfriend and I broke up, and I set up shop in a new home in the San Fernando Valley. Right around that time, I entered a charming phase where I wore embarrassingly small outfits and far too much makeup, dated wildly inappropriate men, and spent a lot of nights at places so Hollywood-y that they were practically parodies of themselves. That particular era in my life also heavily featured personal quirks that—rather fortunately, I think—flew out of my life along with my twenties: quirks like a desire to be awake on the other side of midnight, a willingness to dance on tabletops just because they were there, a penchant for truly atrocious clip-on hair extensions, and a total refusal to take off my eyeliner before going to sleep.

Why such a particular aversion to innocent things like cotton balls and makeup remover? I don't know, but I suspect a crippling case of The Stubborns may have been involved, enhanced by the fact that when you roll in around 3:00 a.m., responsible personal care habits tend to rate fairly low on your list of priorities.

There was many a morning that my roommate was startled by the sight of what resembled a blonde, mildly hungover panda wandering down the hallway.

Now, the whole "sleeping in three pounds of kohl" thing may not be a great idea even when you're twenty-five, but at this point in my life doing a thing like this would be seriously ill-advised. Forgetting to remove my makeup before bed makes my face angry, and my face likes to voice its displeasure by growing an extra wrinkle overnight just out of spite.

These days, it's not about fixing what's broken . . . it's about preventing things from breaking in the first place.

How-To: STOP BEAUTY DISASTERS BEFORE THEY START

It's a fact: putting a little extra effort into daily care and maintenance saves you a ton of time in the long run, just because healthy hair, skin, and nails tend to look more or less A-OK with very little accoutrement.

- Do not go to sleep with your makeup on. Just don't do it. Ever.

- Drink water, and then drink some more water. And then more. I didn't used to be particularly good about this, and now I am, and it is the single thing that has made the biggest difference in how I look (and feel) when I wake up every morning. If you don't love regular old water, try adding lemon juice, cucumber slices, grapefruit wedges, or even a couple of drops of artificial flavor to it; whatever gets it into your body.

- Apply moisturizer and eye cream every single night, no excuses.

- Likewise, if you find that you're occasionally ending the day simply too exhausted to even spend a minute washing your face, keep some cleansing wipes and pre-moistened makeup remover pads in your bedside table so you can barely move a muscle and still go to bed with clean skin.

- Try to get quality rest. Having a baby can seriously disrupt your sleep patterns, so try a lavender-scented eye mask, a sound machine, or a pre-bedtime chamomile tea ritual. Or all three (hey, whatever works).

- Use a shampoo and conditioner that are tailored to your hair's specific needs (color-treated, dry, et cetera), and enhance the effects with a weekly intensive repair mask.

- If you don't have time to get to the salon, keep your fingernails looking neat by filing them and then buffing them lightly to add shine.

Lighten Up

You know how they say that wearing less makeup, choosing fewer accessories, and generally streamlining everything from your wardrobe to your hairstyle makes you look younger?

In my experience, it's true.

I'm usually on autopilot when it comes to applying makeup: I have my routine, and I have the products that I use, and I don't even have to think about it. But every so often it's a good idea to put the autopilot on pause and reevaluate what you're doing, to see if it's really working for you . . . meaning the right-now you.

When I was in college, I wore dark eyeliner both on my top eyelids and on the inner rims of the lower lids, and my boyfriend hated it. I ignored him completely, of course, and went right on applying my makeup exactly how I wanted to. It wasn't until I was pregnant and I found myself wanting to look more "fresh" than "glamorous" that the lower-lid liner went into my drawer, never again to re-emerge once I discovered that while it might have looked edgy and dramatic when I was younger, all it was doing for me now was aging me.

On Saturday morning, I showed up at a fashion event I was hosting wearing nothing more than a touch of shadow and some mascara, and three separate people commented on how rested I looked.

I *never* look rested.

So when three separate people say that I do, I listen.

Also: When you're used to wearing what's really quite a lot of makeup, it can feel strangely uncomfortable to lighten up. It's silly, of course, but it's true: I sometimes like to hide, just a little. Behind liner that evens out my asymmetrical eyes, behind a lipstick that makes it look like I'm pulled-together even when I'm feeling anything but, behind a pair of sunglasses that hides the puffiness, the lines, the fact that I'm so tired so much of the time.

But lately, I've been doing . . . less. It feels simultaneously good and not-good, and I think that's fine. I have a picture in my head of the woman I want to be in twenty years, and she's not a Real Housewife; she's just real. Maybe even a little calm and wise; that would be nice.

I guess I just want to look like myself at the moment, whatever it is that means. I feel like it might be okay. And that might have something to do with realizing that as I get older less is possibly more, but it also might not even be about makeup at all. Maybe it's just about wanting, for whatever reason, to put fewer things between my skin and the world.

TWO-MINUTE NO-TIME NEW MAMA MAKEUP

Oof, do I ever love this beauty routine. You know how a "natural" effect is almost always way harder to create than it looks? Not this one. With just a handful of products—most of which you probably already own—you can go from looking like . . . well, like someone who's just had a baby, to looking fresh as a daisy in (literally) two minutes.

Go ahead, time it.

1. Start with a tinted moisturizer. Even better, go for a BB (or CC) cream that also contains anti-aging and color-correcting ingredients; you'll take care of all your skin's needs in a single step.

2. Give your cheeks a soft flush of color with a blush that suits your skin tone. Skip the sparkly formulas (these can be a little harsh for the daytime), and if your skin is dry, try a cream blush that will blend in seamlessly.

3. Brighten up your eye area by swiping a pale pink or ivory shadow across the entire lid.

4. Apply several coats of a lengthening mascara.

5. Finish with tinted lip balm to simultaneously moisturize and add color to your lips.

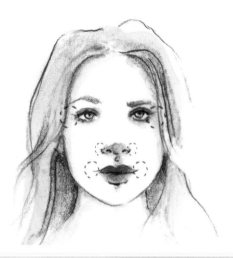

Let's Talk False Eyelashes (Stay with Me Here)

If—and I mean only *if*—you have an extra minute and want to look really spectacular, I have one more suggestion: false eyelashes.

I know, you're all; "Jordan, you loon, false eyelashes are *not* a speedy beauty solution; they're a totally indulgent and ridiculously laborious extra that has absolutely no place in my life right now." But stay with me for a second.

It's true: Until you figure out the process, false eyelashes are a pain . . . but once you get the hang of them, they're on and busy making you look gorgeously wide-awake in seconds. Add them to the No-Time New Mama Beauty Routine just described and they're all you need to take you from day to Date Night. And the total time you spent on your makeup all day long? About three minutes.

MINI FALSE EYELASH TUTORIAL

1. Individual lashes offer the most natural effect . . . but they also make me impatient, so what I go for are cheapie drugstore-brand half-lashes (or full lashes that I've snipped in half); they're way easier to apply than individual lashes or full strips, and I like the lengthening effect of adding lashes to just the outer corners of your eyes.

2. Coat the edge of the lash strip with a thin layer of eyelash adhesive. If you have trouble applying the right amount of glue directly from the tube, try dotting some onto a tissue and gently dragging the edge of the strip through the droplet.

3. Place the halved lash strip at the outer corner of your eye, snuggling it down into your natural lash line so it blends with your real lashes.

4. Finally, tap the lashes gently into place with the tips of your fingers and let them dry.

5. Repeat on the other eye.

LOSE THOSE RED LIPS

I am an enormous proponent of the power of the right red lipstick to instantly make you look awake and amazing. Before my son was born, I'd actually have called red lipstick my "signature" (if I enjoyed saying things like "it's my signature," which I do not).

After he was born? Bye-bye, red. The fact is that babies need to be held a lot, and once you've wiped off smudges of crimson from duckling-soft hair or scrubbed it out of adorable little hats a few times you start thinking, "You know what? Let's just leave that whole red lipstick thing for later, when a child's head isn't in constant close proximity to my face."

Tinted balms are great, but if you find that even those end up decorating your baby's lovely locks, try this trick: Fill in your lips with a nude lip pencil, and then top with a light application of colorless balm (go for a non-glossy formula) to keep them looking and feeling soft. Your color should stay put right where it's supposed to all day long.

When Tired Eyes Are Smiling

You know how new mothers are typically fairly tired human beings? Well, I get to do them one better, because on top of the ordinary "there is a small person in my house who won't let me sleep" thing, I've suffered from a paralyzingly terrible case of chronic insomnia off and on for about a decade now. Sometimes I lie awake all night because of anxiety, sometimes because I have freakishly good hearing and can hear every single thing that happens in the house all night long (from my dog licking his foot over and over and over to the boiler kicking on to my husband breathing), and once it was because I was startled awake at 1:55 a.m. by the words *Jenna von Oÿ*. As in the actress who played the sidekick on *Blossom* about twenty years ago.

Not out loud. In my head. And the weirdness of that event was enough to prevent me from falling back asleep for the remainder of the night.

Sleep disorders, whee!

No, but honestly: It's kind of the worst, and means that I often spend the hours between 1:00 a.m. and 5:00 a.m. carrying my pillow pathetically from room to room in an effort to find a magical sleep spot and doing weird things like eating bananas and opening random cabinets to see whether a small, helpful person might be waiting inside to tell me exactly what I need to do in order to finally pass out.

It also means that I frequently have a case of The Under-Eye Bags to rival your resident bloodhound's.

But the fact that I prefer to not look like a zombie (even if I feel like one) also means that I've come up with a handful of quick tips for faking a wide-awake appearance rather well. And if you're a new mother, insomniac or no, these are tips that I suspect might come in handy from time to time.

- Store your under-eye cream either in the refrigerator or next to a drafty window; the cooling effect will help to wake you up in seconds.

- Finish your morning shower with a one-second blast of freezing water. Sounds terrible; it's actually amazing. If you have no time to shower, try soaking a washcloth in ice water and pressing it to your face for a few moments.

- Apply a subtle highlighter or a swipe of pale shadow to the inner corners of your eyes (just avoid anything too sparkly or metallic, which can be harsh and aging).

- Pick up a nude-toned eyeliner and lightly rim the inside of the lower lid; this will pull out the redness and make your eyes look more wide-open.

- Use an eyelash curler followed by a lengthening mascara, concentrating on the lashes at the outer edges of your eyes.

One Last Thing about Beauty and Balance

Earlier in this chapter I talked about growing up a bit, and in the process learning that (ba da dum!) my self-worth isn't actually tied to my ability to apply liquid liner before a trip to CVS . . . and I was joking, of course.

But also—of course—not joking, not exactly.

I write often about the time in my life when I lived in Los Angeles and was very, very sad because it still takes me by surprise: the realization that the person I was then and the person I am now are one and the same. It was a time in my life when I didn't like the story that my eyes told when I looked into the mirror, and so I painted my face over and over, covering up my skin so that it would tell me something different. Lie for me.

I think about that time often because it was a time when I spent an enormous amount of energy trying to distract myself and everyone around me from what was inside, which felt like nothing at all. I was terrified of ending up as nothing more than a cautionary tale of what happens to young girls who move to Hollywood to become actresses, and I felt very strongly that that was exactly where my story was headed.

Eventually I did "fail," if you want to call it that (because that's certainly how it felt): I was fired from a television show that I had helped to create and had worked on developing for over a year—a show that everyone had called my "big break"—then fired by my fancy new manager who had taken me on solely because of that show, and then finally fired by my agent of over a decade. And an actor without an agent is an actor in serious trouble.

I failed, and it was possibly the best thing that ever happened to me.

Losing what I thought I wanted was what finally let me *let go* . . . and, partially because I wanted to and mostly because I had no other alternative, I went flying off in another direction entirely—a direction that brought me to a life that makes me happy in ways that I would never even have imagined way back when I was driving endlessly up and down the California coastline. Am I happier because I settled down into a career that I loved? Because of my husband and child? Because I live in a home that's mine, and that has a garden where I can grow tomatoes? It's all of those things, and also nothing quite so simple; it was the switch that happened inside—the return to a lesson that I learned long ago, and then forgot somewhere along the way—that made finding those things even possible.

I make steaks and asparagus almost every week, and when I collapse into bed each night I don't hear the sounds of seagulls calling out to each other over an empty beach, but rather the sounds of my family—my husband turning magazine pages downstairs, my dogs padding around on a hunt for an errant kernel of popcorn, my son's deep, even breaths. All that time I spent waiting for my turn—all that "almost" time—was replaced by the Right Now.

In the space of a decade, things—everything, really—changed, and is changing even now. But still, sometimes I remember that girl who spent a summer in Malibu putting her hair up and then back down again, and I can't help but wonder whether the things I write about, *care* about—ways to make your home and your life beautiful in small, easy ways—have any real place in days that are so full to the brim with family and work and responsibilities that really, honestly need to be addressed before attention can be paid to something as small—as meaningless, in the scheme of it all—as a pretty shade of lipstick, or a hairdo.

The answer, of course, is that these small things are not meaningless. The ways in which we choose to add beauty to our lives are valuable beyond measure, and they are not about any one tip or piece of makeup or article of clothing: They are about finding what matters to you, what makes you feel lovely, and then making those unique, cherished things a part of your world.

It is important to make time for the things that make you feel like your weird, wonderful self, whatever they may be.

But more than anything, more than it all, it's important to know this: your life, your self, exactly as it is:

Is beautiful.

When I was thirteen years old and wearing Salvation Army pajamas and glitter eye shadow to school, I was saying something very important without even knowing it; something that I forgot as the years went on and that I lost sight of entirely during that summer in Malibu. Beauty isn't about a picture that you have in your head that you think will bring you to a place that's brighter, better, happier than the place you are right now; it's about saying out loud what makes you feel good, and then being brave enough to let the world see what makes you tick. It was a great lesson for a teenager to learn, and a lesson I had to re-teach myself many years later.

I'm thirty-two now. My skin is older; my stomach is looser; my hair is wilder because my straightening iron only gets turned on when tiny hands aren't around to touch it. And yet I feel beautiful. Right here, sitting at my dining room table in front of my computer, wearing clothes that don't match, my eyeglasses pushed up on my head, my bangs doing something strange and disobedient.

I feel beautiful just as I am, and it's such a surprise.

I used to wear mascara because it was a thing that I could use to pretend to be someone strong and lovely when inside I felt anything but. My face matches my heart; it always has, for better or for worse. But now the story the mirror tells is the story of my life and my family and the things that we have built together, and I put on mascara just because I like to.

"Just because" is reason enough sometimes. And the splashes of color that I sprinkle over each day: Now they're just little additions to a life that's mine, and that's real, and that I'm actually *living*—not one that I'm dreaming of while watching the waves pull back into the sea.

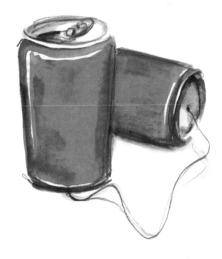

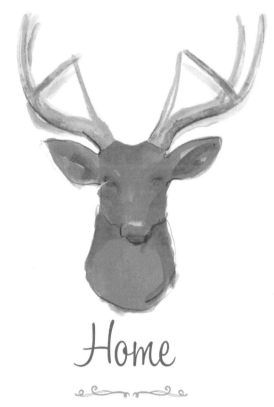

Home

(Babies Throw Up a Lot, but You Still Probably Need to Own a Couch)

Your Family, Your Life, Your Space

I have what could generously be termed "a mild couch fixation," and what could more accurately be called "a total obsession bordering on the crazy-pants that makes my husband occasionally consider abandoning me in the woods to be raised by a deer family rather than continue living with a manic couch—purchasing looney tune for one more minute."

You could say I've bought a few couches in my day.

Fortunately, this little couch-buying problem of mine hasn't really had a negative impact on anyone except for Kendrick (who has toted a couch up and down several flights of stairs an average of once every six months for the bulk of our seven-year relationship). I mean, the majority of the couches that I've owned over the years have been hand-me-downs or secondhand buys, so it's not like I was throwing us into the poorhouse; we're talking an average of a hundred bucks a pop. And moving beyond the nitty-gritties of cash flow into the spiritual realm for just a moment, I would like to make sure you're aware that the three boys who showed up at my apartment to divest me of one of my couches—intensely, almost impressively stoned individuals who walked through our front door and evaluated my couch for approximately half a second before announcing that they were going to cut off its legs and take it with them to a rave—were pretty psyched about the whole situation, so there you go: couch karma.

My first post-college couch was a white, slipcovered cutie-pie from Ikea that (I thought) elevated my very first apartment back in Los Angeles from featureless box to glam single-lady dwelling. It was exactly the same couch that every other person I knew owned, except mine was snow white. Why white, you ask? Because I enjoy living dangerously, because I had convinced myself that a person who harbored a strong affection for Two Buck Chuck should drink that Chuck while sitting on white furniture, and because I had not yet internalized the lesson that we will cover in the section of this chapter, "I Never Want to Own Anything White Ever Again in My Life, Ever." I was over-the-moon about that couch for a hot minute, and then it turned yellow, developed a less-than-desirable patina that I suspect was the offspring of Two-Buck Chuck droplets and Los Angeles smog, and basically disintegrated.

After my white sofa died an unglamorous death, I moved on to a streamlined brown couch that I thought was so extremely chic that it could more accurately be called "espresso" . . . but then ended up looking not-so-cute in the aftermath of an apparently exhausting cross-country trip during which I have to assume that all three of the very large movers I hired to help me get from L.A. to New York sat on it, slept on it, and took it to parties and gave it tequila shots.

Chic Espresso Couch was followed by a cozy striped hand-me-down from my parents that looked vaguely like a reject from the Big Apple Circus and that I hear ended its life as the centerpiece of a rave. Next came a fairly amazing powder-blue custom job that I bought from a nice old lady who lived a couple of blocks away from us on the Upper East Side and that I adored, cherished, and petted like a beloved, powder-blue golden retriever until I discovered that sitting on it felt like riding on a bushel of cement. Finally there was Chic Espresso Couch #2, which was just the ticket for a short while, after which we spontaneously grew a second dog and a human child and realized that, diminutively elegant as the thing was, exactly one-fifth of our family was able to comfortably fit on it at one time.

Last of all came the couch we own now: the very first for-real, grown-up (by which I mean horrendously expensive and previously owned by no one else) couch I have ever bought. It is the couch of my dreams, and I mean that literally: I have dreamed about it because I am the kind of person who dreams about couches.

It's approximately the size of Texas, has a chaise lounge section that I claimed as my own within moments of its arrival, and when my husband and I sit down on it together to watch a movie or show I don't even know that he *exists* . . . and that is an awesome thing, because at this particular juncture in my life, floating on my own personal couch boat and concentrating on the intricacies of *The Bachelor* takes priority over snuggling. It's also already looking a little run-down thanks to my dog's determination to spend a minimum of ten hours per day perched on the back cushion (only the one on the left, of course, so as to maximize asymmetry), and the color isn't exactly what I thought it would be when I looked at the swatch in the store . . . and ask me if I care?

I do not.

I love it, smooshy cushions, not-exactly-the-color-I-expected fabric and all.

And I love it not because it is a Style-Expert Approved couch, all ready and waiting for its *Elle Decor* pictorial. I love it because when I lay in my little chaise lounge corner my son curls up in the crook of my arm, my dogs settle down around my feet, and my husband stretches out across the rest of it, and when a sippy cup gets spilled or a dog drools or some Chinese food ends up where it shouldn't be . . . guess what?

It's microfiber, bitches. And drool comes off of it like nobody's business.

It's not a couch for the style pages; it's a couch for my *life*.

Why am I starting a chapter of this book in which I'm ostensibly offering up tips to pull together your own home with a rundown of Sort-Of Couch Failures? Because the point of it all isn't getting an A+ in Home Decor class . . . the point of it all is making the world that you and your family inhabit *yours*. Creating a beautiful home, a home that you adore (and pulling your home together *is* an act of creation) isn't about getting things perfectly all the time, or even most of the time. It's about surrounding yourself with a collection of things that remind you of the people and places that you love the most. That have stories. That are *alive*, and that aren't what some guy on HGTV told you that you should like, but are rather what inspire you and make you feel like you're right where you want to be.

Right now, as I sit in my living room typing these words, I'm surrounded by:

- A midcentury-style coffee table that I bought for a 1950s-themed segment of my home décor show, and that I ended up having to hire someone to assemble because it just wasn't going to happen on my watch;
- A 1970s rocker-and-ottoman set that I found in a charity thrift store and that, despite all Google-sourced evidence to the contrary, I am absolutely convinced is worth a small fortune;
- Four clear plastic chairs that I bought at Ikea because I'm obsessed with Philippe Starck Ghost Chairs and will not be able to afford them in this lifetime; and
- An upright piano that I found at the Salvation Army on Eleventh Avenue, dragged up to the suburbs, and painted black because that seemed like the best way to disguise the fact that the thing is really kind of a piece of junk.

And I love it all. Because it's mine, because it's real, and because it tells a story . . . and the story that it tells is the story of my life, and my family's lives, and the things that we have built together.

The point of this chapter isn't how to get it "right" . . . it's how to get it right for *you*. These are tips, ideas, and things that have worked (or not worked) for me, but that's all they are—suggestions. Take from it what you like, leave what you don't, and remember that when it comes down to it, you are the boss of you, and you are the boss of your home. And if you want to spray-paint your old dining room set neon green and re-cover the seats of the chairs with cow-print fabric (which sounds fantastic, just saying), that's what you should do. What's the worst thing that can happen? You don't like it?

Big deal.

It's just decoration. And it should be fun.

Inspiration Boards and Getting Started

I blame my parents for everything.

And today I'm going to blame them for the fact that despite my knee-jerk aversion to the very term "inspiration board," that's exactly what I'm going to tell you that I think you should make before you purchase even one more tiny little thing with which to decorate your home.

When I was twelve years old and into wearing pajamas to school, my parents may have been slightly leery of their only child's judgment, but they never said a word. In fact, from what I could tell they were totally A-OK with my sartorial experimenta-tion—it was all in the service of personal expression. When, in ninth grade, I decided that I was a witch and filled my bedroom with pentagrams, crystal balls, and incense burners, and then headed to math class decked out in floor-length tie-dyed gowns with sleeves so enormous that they trailed on the ground, same thing: fine by them.

And when I was fifteen and decided to wallpaper the cabinets in my bedroom from top to bottom with a collage of everything that a sixteen-year-old might think is cool, they handed me a bunch of double-sided tape and let me do my thing.

And so I blame my parents for it all—the hot pink, gold-antlered deer head sitting in my sunroom, the mild fixation on animal prints, the tendency to adorn thrift store finds with gold-leaf paint . . .

Everything.

Back to those collage-wallpapered bedroom cabinets, though, because they were *amazing*. My friends and I decorated them with photographs that we'd taken of each other, of the fire escapes and Central Park pathways and apartment stoops that were the backdrops of our lives, and of boys we went on dates with and boys who didn't even know our names, and then we accessorized it all with postage stamps, stickers, magazine pictorials, and anything else we could think of. We had this one black-and-white shot of a teacher we all had a crush on, and we surrounded it with photos of all of us gazing in his direction, complete with heart-shaped cutout thought bubbles. Later on, this very same teacher wrote me a recommendation letter that I suspect very strongly was a major factor in my admission to college, so there you go: wish fulfillment. Sort of.

I suppose you could call that wall my very first inspiration board.

Let's take a step back, though, because if you're anything like me I can feel you rolling your eyes from all the way over here. I mean . . . am I really advocating that fully-grown adults who theoretically have stuff to do like, oh, I don't know, work at jobs and make money and cook dinner and raise actual human people spend their time making *inspiration boards*?

Really?

But you're going to have to bear with me here, because if I am suggesting that you get yourself involved with things like fabric swatches and glue sticks, you better believe I have a good reason for it.

No exaggeration: Creating a realistic, goal-oriented inspiration board is my

Number One trick for pulling together a space that you love without spending so much money that you fall into a pit of not-quite-right-coffee-table-owning regret. Done right, an inspiration board can help you to seamlessly incorporate the items that you already own into the room of your dreams, ultimately ending up with a space that's both stunningly beautiful and uniquely your own.

Shall we discuss? Let's focus on the nursery for now, but really, this technique can (and, I think, should) be applied to any room you'd like to rehab.

How-To: CREATE AN INSPIRATION BOARD

1. So you may be starting from scratch, but chances are you already own at least a couple of pieces of furniture or tchotchkes that you'd really like to include . . . so the first thing to do when creating an inspiration board is to assess the space in question and make a list of the items that you definitely want to keep. These can include furnishings that you don't want to replace, a wall color that you're in love with, or an antique that you absolutely adore. Anything goes, so long as you're honest and realistic about what you want to hold on to—and what you're willing to let go of.

2. Next, decide what medium makes the most sense for you. There are two basic ways to create an inspiration board:

   A. (SORT OF) HIGH-TECH. Use a website or program that allows you to cut and paste uploaded photos or images you clip from the Web onto a digital composite board. This is what I do, mostly because once you get the hang of it, it's easy. But I also love how the finished product looks; it all makes me feel very interior designer-y and fancy.

   B. MAJORLY LOW-TECH. Break out the paper or posterboard and just glue on pictures cut out of magazines, fabric swatches, and photographs.

3. Start your inspiration board with clipped images of items that resemble the things that you already decided that you didn't want to part with back

in step 1. Remember, however, that these representations *don't have to be exact*: if you have a gray couch but can't find a picture of a gray couch, just find a gray square that's more or less the right shade; if you have a blue rug, a blue circle cut from a magazine works just fine. You get the idea.

4. Arrange the images of your existing pieces on the board to serve as a starting point, remembering to keep in mind the general dimensions and limitations of the space you're working with. Also remember that you can always change their position later on—nothing is set in stone.

5. Now's the fun part: Start filling out the board with images—colors, patterns, items—that you love. A really cool chair, an amazing shade of hot pink, a tiger-print pillow . . . anything goes. Move the images around, adding and subtracting, until you find an arrangement that feels right.

The goal: To arrive at a space that's both filled with the kinds of things that make you happy and that's visually coherent.

Let's say that you already own a white crib, some silver end tables, and a couple of teal lamps. Let's also say that you are considering buying a small green pillow shaped like an alien robot.

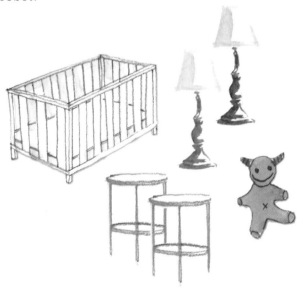

A few minutes of playing around with your inspiration board might show you that you like the way a peach rug and a dark leather rocker warms up the pieces you already own, but that you should maybe skip picking up a little pillow friend in that exact shade, adorable though he may be.

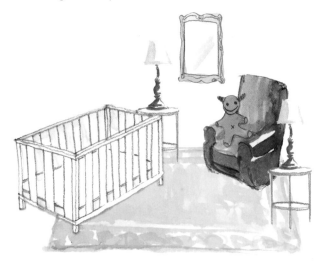

Alternatively, let's say that you or your child have a serious thing for small char-treuse creatures with horns, and that what you really would like to do is decorate around that particular item.

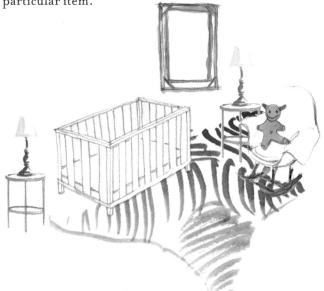

There you go. Aren't you glad that you now know that it would be a really good idea to hunt for a zebra rug on your next outing?

I'm glad, too.

The point of all this: Instead of going to a department store and buying a roomful of furniture and decorative items all at once because they're right there in front of you, all matchy-matchy and pre-approved by whoever puts together store displays, an inspiration board helps you to figure out what colors and patterns and general styles you want to go for . . . so you can head to your local thrift store, flea market, or discount furniture shop with those starting points in mind. Not only do you save money, you end up with a space that's 100 percent "you" from top to bottom.

And *that's* what I call style.

Small Spaces and Small People

One night way back in February 2007, my high school friend Jake and I were playing around on MySpace and he showed me the page of a Brooklyn-based indie band whose lead singer had been a couple of years behind us at school. I friend-requested the band just for fun, the keyboardist sent me a message asking me to come to one of their shows, and a few weeks later, during a break in their tour schedule, he came out to visit me in Los Angeles. We road-tripped to Las Vegas, and ended up at a pawnshop at three in the morning in search of an engagement ring.

We set a wedding date for the following summer, and I decided that I should probably move back to New York City so that I could get to know my new fiancé.

By May, I had packed up or sold everything I owned and flown back across the country with my (now "our") one-eyed shih tzu. We found a tiny one-bedroom apartment in Hell's Kitchen, just a couple of blocks away from Times Square, and made it home with a mosaic-topped coffee table we picked up at the Salvation Army, my parents' Big Apple Circus couch, and a turquoise dresser with crystal handles that I'd found on Craigslist practically for free because it was half-broken, but that I'd dragged up to our apartment anyway just because I liked the color so much.

The apartment was so small that we had to sit on the bed in order to open the closet doors or dresser drawers, and in the summers we crawled out through the kitchen window and ate slices of pizza on the fire escape, just to have a little extra space. On December 31, we climbed up onto the roof of our building and watched as the Times Square ball dropped into the new year.

After two years of a bathroom you could barely turn around in and a two-burner stove and a bed that was too big for our bedroom but still way too small for the two of us (plus dog), we decided to upgrade to an apartment on the Upper East Side that was easily twice the size of our Hell's Kitchen place. It was 750 whole square feet, and it even had a *second bedroom* (or, more accurately, a wide-ish section of the hallway that ran between the living room and the actual bedroom). And it was rent-controlled. I thought I had up and discovered my own personal paradise, and immediately began making plans to stay there forever and ever.

After we'd been living in that apartment for a year or so, we started thinking it might be nice to have a baby. Why not?! We were in love, we had health insurance, and by New York City standards we were practically living in a mansion. Sure, we wouldn't have tons and tons of space, and sure, we didn't know exactly where those things (like car seats and strollers and cribs) that we'd heard come along with a baby might go, but big deal. We'd just be all awesomely chilled-out and easygoing and make it work with the space we had.

Except I forgot one small detail: I am not awesomely chilled-out and easygoing. Like, ever.

The second I found out I was pregnant, which was about two seconds after we decided that it might be okay to start trying, I reacted in the only way that made sense to me: by ordering random Ikea cabinets off the Internet and making my husband assemble them *right now*. I also moved chairs from one room to another, stood in front of our single closet and worried a bunch about how small it was, and then cried because there was no countertop in our kitchen, and I didn't know where the bottle drying thing was going to go.

And then I decided to pretend to be an actual grown-up human being who was capable of caring for the infant who was going to arrive in about nine months whether we were ready for him or not, and sat down with a pen and some paper to figure out how, exactly, we'd make our apartment make sense for a baby.

And guess what?

It worked out just fine.

It was actually pretty adorable.

How-To: SET UP A NURSERY IN A SMALL SPACE

Remember that inspiration board that we talked about a few pages back? This is a really good time to get over the fact that it sounds tremendously silly and actually do it, because (especially if you're working with budget and/or space constraints) an inspiration board is going to make your life a whole lot easier when it comes to actually purchasing the pieces you need.

If "The Nursery" is actually "A Corner of Your Bedroom":

• Make sure that the style you choose for the major pieces blends with the style of the rest of the room. A clean, contemporary palette of layered whites and creams is always pretty, and you can add in splashes of the colors you've used elsewhere in the room to add interest.

• An area rug can help to separate out the nursery space from the rest of the room. Just make sure to go for a rug that's easy to clean (and Scotchgard that baby), because trust me: You will have the occasional changing table-related disaster, and it will be bad.

- Choose pieces that pull double-duty, like a crib with a changing station that attaches to the top rails (thereby eliminating the need for a separate changing table) or a storage ottoman that can be used both for seating and for holding extra crib sheets.

- Go for space-saving styles. We picked up a "snuggle nest" that went right between us in our own bed instead of a bassinet, and chose a small vibrating baby seat rather than a large swing that would have taken up half of our living room.

- Get creative with storage: Pick up baskets that fit under the crib to store things like towels and blankets. Stash toys and books in pretty storage cubes that easily blend with your décor style, and pick up a diaper caddy to organize your wipes, lotions, and diapers.

- Install shelving units and decorative wall boxes to display mementos; these let you show off books, toys, and photos without taking up floor or counter-top space.

> **Remember: Don't go overboard with the buying. A newborn needs about one-eighteenth of the things that stores will tell you that they need when you're putting together a registry.**

SMALL SPACE STORAGE

You know what one of the strangest things about moving from Tiny Apartment to Small Apartment (and then, a couple of years later, to Small House) was? How weird-quickly our stuff expanded to fill our brand-new (and, we had thought, much larger) space. And we're talking about *the same stuff*. Maybe the movers fed our furniture Twinkies the entire trip or maybe a furniture elf arrived in the night and put our dining room table under a spell that caused it to magically expand, but either way: Despite the actual square footage of my surroundings, I have somehow managed to spend most of my life not having enough room for stuff.

Which might mean that I have too much stuff.

But because few things make me crazier than clutter, it also means that I've gotten extremely good at putting all this stuff away.

How-To: SMALL-SPACE STORAGE

DO A SEASONAL SWAP-OUT. The first thing you have to do is commit to spending a little time every few months taking every single non-seasonally-appropriate item out of your closet and packing it away. I keep one storage bag under my bed, as well as a bunch of big clear plastic boxes in an easy-to-access part of our basement.

CLEAR OUT THE SPECIAL ITEMS. Keep all the pieces that you definitely want to hold onto but only wear once in a blue moon (gowns, ski jackets, your mother's amazing-but-not-really-wearable 1970s jumpsuit) out of your primary closet area, so that you don't have to sift through them every morning while on the hunt for something you can actually put on to head to Dunkin' Donuts.

FIND STORAGE SPOTS EVERYWHERE. There is not a single nook or cranny in our house that hasn't been called into action. Sheets are kept in soft zip-up boxes under our son's crib, the backs of doors hold shoes, coat racks in corners store purses and scarves . . . even the little hidden spot between our wardrobe and the wall holds my computer bag and camera tripod. Hunt down all those small spaces. I promise, they add up to quite a lot.

LOOK FOR WAYS TO CREATE PRETTY DISPLAYS. Some stuff—like, say, extra pillowcases—should really be tucked away out of sight both because it's messy-looking, and because you don't need it readily accessible at all times. But other things—like shoes, purses, and jewelry—can sometimes be left right out in plain view; don't waste valuable storage space on items that can be repurposed as décor.

DISPLAY IDEAS

A. Hang hooks on your wall and use them to create a display of your nicest purses (use the same principles for creating a gallery wall; see page 94).

B. If you have a gorgeous shoe collection, pick up a shoe storage bench and let it double up as an end table, a TV table, or even (why not?) a coffee table.

C. Find interesting ways to display your jewelry:

- Push tacks into a board to create a display for your prettiest pieces

- Use a pretty overdoor hook to hang necklaces

- Set a beautiful cake plate on your vanity to display your bangles; the plate provides extra surface area and the height creates visual interest

- Get creative with found objects: Sculptures and knickknacks from flea markets and thrift stores can easily be called into action as jewelry displays

BABIES ARE CUTE,
BUT YOURS IS THE CUTEST

My husband and I have always been pretty big on taking photographs, but we hit some next-level action when our son was born. I mean, man, babies are cute. And if you happen to have a real live baby sitting right there in your house next to you, chances are you're going to want to take a photo or forty thousand of it. But if you're living in a smallish space (and even if you're not), there are only so many surfaces upon which one can perch a photo frame.

For those who've become a little trigger-happy with the camera, here's an easy, space-saving (and chic) solution: a gallery wall.

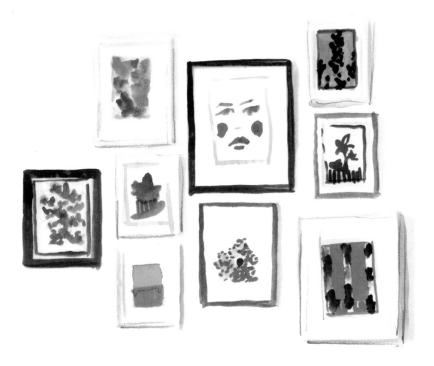

DIY GALLERY WALL

1. Start with an odd number of framed family photos (I like using mismatched frames in the same color family—all white, all gold, et cetera—but whatever works for you).

2. Choose the wall where you're going to place your gallery.

3. Measure that wall to find its exact center. That's the spot where you *don't* want to put a photo. Why? Because placing a picture in the exact center of the wall draws too much focus to that one image, and your goal is to keep the eye moving across all of your adorable shots.

4. You can create paper templates of your frames and use some tape to play around with the orientation of the frames before actually picking up the hammer and nails . . . but I'm impatient, so I simply go ahead and hang the first photo just to the side of the wall's center and then move outward from there, placing frames wherever seems like a good spot.

I Never Want to Own Anything White Ever Again in My Life, Ever (Stain Removal Tips)

In today's Earth-Shattering News: There is a lot of gross stuff that goes on when you're dealing with a human being who is not yet in possession of a reliably functional digestive system.

All right, let's do it.
Let's talk about the gross stuff.

I try to avoid all those bodily-function conversations that very naturally come along with parenthood on Ramshackle Glam because . . . well, (a) I know not everyone who reads the site is a parent, and I'm not sure I would have loved reading about this stuff pre-baby arrival, and (b) gross. It's just really gross.

But I'm going to tell you what just happened to me this morning, again for a couple of reasons:

1. Those of you who aren't yet parents may be one day, and preparation is half the battle, blah blah blah . . .
2. I need sympathy.

Look, I'm not new to the world of projectile vomiting. I went to college, too.

But today was something special.

Because there was an incident in the very early morning (requiring replacement of onesie, sheets, and assorted stuffed animals), and then a situation in the late morning (requiring two parental clothing changes, a full kitchen Fantastik-ing, and the corralling of dogs who appear to view vomit as a five-star meal—I told you this was gross, I'm sorry) . . . and then I drove Kendrick to work, and THREE SECONDS after I drove away there was an incident in the car.

Car seats are like little *Battlestar Galacticas*, that's how hard they are to assemble. And all that assembly means: straps. And buttons. And bolts.

You know what sucks to clean? Straps and buttons and bolts.

Anyway, it's all fine now. Every creature and piece of clothing and button and bolt in the house is happy, at least passably healthy, and either clean or sitting in a bowl of hot water, soaking.

Oh, except for me. I am *disgusting*.

Now that we've covered the fact that being a parent goes hand-in-hand with the occasional very messy incident, I have some excellent news, and the news is that I'm going to share a secret with you:

I am an actual card-carrying wizard when it comes to getting stuff out of stuff. I'm basically a miracle.

Oh, I'm serious.

It all started with a glass of wine, and a nicer shirt than my husband and I could afford. The shirt didn't belong to *us* . . . it belonged to our very stylish downstairs neighbor, Stephen, who had come over for a drink only to discover that his hostess (me) was possessed of a singular capacity for upending glasses of red liquid directly onto her guests.

His shirt was really nice, guys. I freaked out. And in about five seconds flat I had him standing in our living room stripped naked (from the waist up, at least) while I frantically scrubbed at his shirt in the bathroom.

It was then that I discovered The Process.

And because you have a child, and are about to learn just how very treacherous life with a child can be if you choose to continue ingesting liquids that are not clear (up to you; just saying, white wine's white for a reason), I'm going to share it with you.

Let's talk completely unscientific stain-removal methods.

How-to: GET OUT THAT STAIN LIKE A WIZARD

1. The first thing you need to do is soak the stained area with water*. If it's an article of clothing we're dealing with, get it under the tap. If it's a carpet or upholstered furniture, start ferrying over enormous handfuls of wet paper towels. Call a procession line into action if necessary. Yell at people. Do what you have to do, because the most important thing is that you get it done *fast*.

2. Next, throw a little of whatever soap is handy onto the stain (I usually just use whatever's sitting right next to the sink).

3. Once the stained area is wet and soapy, rub the fabric against itself (or rub the paper towels against the carpet/furniture). Do not be gentle; be awesome.

4. Rinse. If the stain is still lingering, add more soap and water and rub the fabric against itself again, and then repeat as necessary until the stain has been vanquished from your life forever.

It's not rocket science and I'm sure Martha wouldn't approve, but I swear: it works every time.

* Obviously this does not apply to delicate fabrics like silk. Please do not water your silk. Also, please don't buy silk blouses if you have a newborn.

Oh My God, Your Dogs Are
Going to Make You So Angry

The chances that I was going to be a next-level hormonal basket case when I was pregnant were about 50,000 percent, so it kind of stunned my husband and me when, about a week after the test came up positive, we realized that I had yet to have an emotional breakdown of any real significance. I mean, I'd been pregnant for *seven whole days*! That is a lot of days. It was quite clear to me that I had been instantly transformed by the miracle of pregnancy into an awe-inspiring paragon of calm the likes of which the world had rarely seen, and that I was going to drift through the coming months so glowy and peaceful that I would inspire those around me to comment on my glowy peacefulness in the kinds of hushed, reverent tones reserved for saints and Angelina Jolie. How lovely.

Oh, but then.

Let me start by saying that I adore my dogs. Lucy came first, a teeny-tiny ball of sweetness and fluff that barreled through my front door—a gift from an ex-boyfriend—and straight into my heart. She instantly became the object of my obsession, traveled with me everywhere I went, and slept right next to me, tucked up under the sheets. When the man who later became my husband arrived on the scene and began taking up valuable space in what she very obviously considered "her" bed, she grumbled until it became clear to all parties involved that this was not a fight that he was going to win. Ever.

Virgil arrived on Christmas Eve a few years later. We opened his carrying crate, and he immediately ran into our bedroom, put his head in my boot, and peed.

He was a present from my husband, who certainly meant well . . . but did not realize that his gift was about to keep us up all night, every night for months, thereby creating some truly spectacular marital strife that, quite fortunately, seemed to have the happy effect of getting the "IT'S YOUR TURN TO DEAL WITH IT" argument out of our system. By the time a for-real infant was the thing keeping us up all night we'd both been so emotionally beaten-down by our insane dog that we were more or less over the whole "sleeping" thing and handled it rather well, actually.

Anyway, my dogs are very cute and I love them.

But the second I got pregnant, they showed their true colors, and their true colors are "asshole" ones.

That's right, I called my dogs assholes. Cuteness and love aside, they seriously are. Yours probably are, too. And if you don't have dogs: everyone else's dogs? Assholes. You know what I'm talking about.

Back to about a week after we found out I was pregnant. I came home from a long day of work, sort of dramatically crashed through our front door, and announced to my husband (with illustrative hand-flutter motions) that he needed to get out of the way so that I could proceed directly to the bedroom—no hugs, no kisses, no human communication, thanks—and pass out. (Obviously I said all this in a very peaceful and glowy way.) Out of my way he went, because he is nice and also because he is smart, and I hand-fluttered my way into the bedroom. . . .

Only to discover a very wet bed and a very guilty-looking Virgil sitting right there on the quilt next to his Circle of Destruction.

You guys, I was *really* tired. And I'm usually an enormous complainer when I'm tired and someone or something is preventing me from sleeping, but now I was tired *and* newly pregnant, and that combination made me pretty confident that I had an excuse to go straight from "Mildly Irritating Whining" into "Full-Scale Meltdown, DEFCON 1."

And so I collapsed onto the floor.

I spent the next half hour sort of shuffling around the apartment and wailing (this, of course, to ensure that my husband was aware of just exactly how upset I was) and doing very little to actually rectify the situation. Eventually we managed to drag the sheets off the bed and pile them into the bathtub, where they would await a morning trip to the local laundromat. I declared despairingly that they would never be clean again. My husband gave me a hug. We put our other set of sheets on the bed. I wailed a little more. My husband gently suggested that I might like to stop wailing and go to sleep. By this point I sort of wanted to watch *Entourage* instead, but decided that he was probably right.

Except I wanted a glass of water first.

So I went to the kitchen, got my water, went back into the bedroom . . .

And Virgil had done it again. On the only other set of sheets that we owned.

In the minutes that followed I put on a performance of such emotional intensity that I honestly have very little recollection of it, but the sum total is that I ended up flat on my back on the floor wailing "WE HAVE NOTHING," because the fact that we had no more sheets for the bed had made me absolutely positive that not only was I never going to be able to sleep again in my life, but that we were also going to be terrible, non-sheet-having parents. And our dog was probably going to pee on our baby.

About nine months after The Pee Heard Round the World, both Lucy and Virgil began preparing for their intensive study in the field of Baby Waking-Up. As of the writing of this book, they have achieved such excellence in this pursuit that they now need nothing more than to watch a leaf gently drift from the tree in our backyard toward the soft grass waiting below to propel them into a round of barking so ear-shattering that not only do they wake up our baby, they wake up all the babies, every-where.

On the plus side, they have also taught our son how to rub his face against our living room rug for a really excellent DIY scratching session, so there's that.

How-To: INTRO YOUR FUR BABIES TO YOUR HUMAN BABY

While I was in the hospital and for a few days afterward, Lucy and Virgil stayed with my parents to give our new arrival a little more space, but we knew that the day when all of the small creatures in our life were going to meet was on the horizon. The thought of introducing our defenseless little newborn to our barky, licky, crazy dogs turned me into a major stressball, and so I armed myself with a ton of Internet research that I can summarize as follows:

"When your dogs meet your baby, they should definitely be on leashes. Do not ever have your dogs on leashes when they meet your baby."

Suffice it to say the experts are conflicted on this topic. But the system that we cobbled together ended working out pretty well.

WHEN DOGGIES MET BABY: OUR PROCESS

1. First, we sent our son's hospital clothing home with my parents so that Lucy and Virgil could theoretically familiarize themselves with his scent prior to actually meeting him. Now, the way my dogs work is that when asked to do something they look at the person making the request as if they are singing the Swedish National Anthem and asking them to join in the fun, so it didn't surprise anyone at all when my parents' request that they sniff the baby's clothing was rewarded with the exact same response that I get when I ask them to do anything, ever: blank stare.

2. Next, we created a "calm" environment for our dogs to come home to. ("Calm" is in quotation marks because our dogs operate on the Losing Their Shit end of the Excitement Scale at every moment in their lives that they are not actually unconscious.)

3. When Lucy and Virgil arrived at our apartment, we made an enormous fuss

over them: kisses, hugs, belly scratches, et cetera. This part was nice.

4. For the actual Baby Introduction, we allowed them into the room with our son one at a time and let them "discover" him on their own. Each dog sniffed him for approximately an eighteenth of a second before heading off in search of something much more fun than a week-old baby.

5. Finally, we rewarded them for not eating our child with something called "bully sticks," which are six-inch-long brown twig-like things that look like beef jerky but are actually dried-out bull penises. These charming treats are also known as "pizzles," and when chewed slowly decompose into a gelatinous white ball that adheres itself to things like carpets and my feet. They are disgusting on an almost incomprehensible level, which is why they are a New Baby Special, and that is it.

Anyway, about five minutes after Dogs met Baby, all three were so over it that they were literally snoring. To me, that's a successful introduction if I've ever seen one. But as with nearly everything baby-related, what it comes down to is combining logic and basic rules of safety with a healthy dose of instinct: You know your child, and you know your pets, and it's you who will know just how best to introduce them. That said, dogs have a tendency to behave unpredictably when faced with stressful situations (like the presence of another living thing that is exactly their size and may or may not whack them in the face), so err on the side of caution.

And don't forget to give them an extra little belly-scratch when you can; they may be assholes, but they're your babies, too.

Making the Move

I loved our Upper East Side apartment, with its built-in bookshelves and arched doorways and one closet and weird bathroom and no countertop and construction zone just outside. I really did. It was everything a young couple—and then a young family—just starting out on a life together needed. There was a diner that sold the best banana splits I've ever had just twenty feet away, and down the street lived a little puppy named Theodore who was so nervous that he carried his blue stuffed bunny in his mouth everywhere he went. In the summertime we walked down to the East River and drank iced coffees from a street vendor while we watched the boats go by. In the fall, we put on hats and boots and took the dogs to Central Park, where we bought warm pretzels to keep us company on a walk through the fallen leaves. And with the biggest snowfall of the year always came that moment right after it stopped, when the streets were quiet and empty of cars and people and we could run straight down the center of the avenue throwing snowballs, jumping through the drifts, and laughing like kids.

Living there wasn't always easy—and once our son arrived wasn't even close to a picnic—but it was real and wonderful and *us*.

It also couldn't last forever. Eventually, we knew, our son would start crawling and then walking and then running, and those 750 square feet wouldn't be enough to contain him. Or maybe they would.

But we didn't *want* them to.

When I was about eight months pregnant, my husband and I developed a crush on a series of small towns nestled along New York's Hudson River, just about an hour outside the city. We started making day trips to those towns, my husband planting both hands in the small of my back to push me and my stomach up the hills that angled steeply northeast from each town's train station to its Main Street. We compared school systems, peeked into rambling Colonials, heard the sounds of baseball bats cracking in the hot evening air, and started seriously considering what it would be like to abandon the city that had been the backdrop of every single moment we had spent in our life together thus far.

We considered, we explored, we argued and examined and turned over and over, and then—slowly, slowly—we started making our way home.

This Kind of Life

I couldn't sleep last night. We're making an offer on a second house, and while I doubt the owners are going to come down enough to allow us to get it, they might . . . and I am definitely more than a little nervous. It is such a big deal. And I'm scared.

The fact is, of course, that this isn't a decision that we've made quickly, or that we haven't thought through: We've been circling the idea of moving since last winter, and have spent the past year saving up and looking at places. And we are both certain that a move is what we want, both on an emotional level and a logical one: The truth is that we're just not reaping any of the benefits of living in Manhattan these days, and city living is getting in the way of our life more than it's enhancing it. Plus, since we'd have to move to someplace more child-friendly (with, say, a bedroom door, and maybe an elevator so I don't feel so trapped) within a year, we'd be talking about rent prices that are at least equal to, if not more than, the kinds of mortgages we're looking at. And finally, I've lived in the suburbs before—in L.A.—and the way of life was much more to my liking: On a Saturday, I'd rather have friends over to BBQ and hang out at home than do . . . well, anything. The things that we like to do best these days are just not the kinds of things that are worth paying to live in the city for.

Most of all, though, the reason we want to move is that city life is not what we want for our son. I grew up here, and I had a great childhood, but I want something different for him. I want him to have a yard to run around in with Lucy and Virgil. I want him to go fishing on Saturdays with his Dad not because it's a big, special production involving car rentals and long drives, but rather because that's just what they feel like doing. I want to pick up our pumpkin in a patch, not in a grocery store. I want him to have a swing set of his very own.

But it's an enormous change for us, and I'd be lying if I said it wasn't scary. I'm scared that I won't make any friends, or that I won't make friends that are the kinds of friends that I have in my life now (which is to say, real friends rather than friends of convenience). I'm scared that Kendrick and I will fight about stupid things like home repairs and mowing the lawn. I'm scared that we'll move in and suddenly realize that we picked the wrong place, and that we would have been happier if we had moved just one town over, or to another state altogether. And you know something else I'm scared of? I'm scared that one day, a few years from now, my husband will wake up and look at me and at the life that we've built and think, *Is that it? Is that all I get?* I'm scared that he'll think that. I'm scared that I'll think that.

Because these towns, you know, they're so quiet. They don't have all those bright city lights to distract you from what's right there in front of you. And what if, when all the lights go down, it's not enough?

Kendrick has a friend who once said that New York City takes all the basic facets of normal human existence away from you, and then sells them back to you one at a time as luxuries. Want a bathroom that fits more than one person at a time? That'll cost ya. A bedroom door? Five hundred extra per month. Don't even ask about closets; you don't get those unless you work on Wall Street.

And the thing about all this struggle—because living in the city is a struggle; it can be such a great ride, but it's certainly not easy—is that it keeps you dreaming that things will change. One day, you say to yourself, I'll move to Italy and have a yard full of lemon trees. Or maybe I'll buy a place in California, right on the ocean. Or maybe I'll find a gorgeous townhouse in the far reaches of Brooklyn. All you know is that where you are right then isn't where you'll likely stay, and there's something very freeing in that knowledge. You don't know where you'll be, but you know it won't be where you are.

Like many others I know of my generation, I was raised by parents who encouraged me to think that I had all the choices in the world, and all the time in the world to make them. We spent years being told that we could do anything, be anything—even our liberal arts curriculums let us play around in various fields for years before choosing a major, if we ever had to at all.

And that's great. It is, it's a wonderful thing—a *privilege*—to feel that you can do anything . . . but it also makes it really hard to finally choose what you want to do. Why should I marry this amazing guy when I've never even been to Asia yet? My even-more-perfect man might be waiting there for me. Why should I accept this pretty cool job offer when I haven't even tested the waters in these five other career paths? I might like something else better. Why should I move to this one town, when there are so many other places in the world that might make the perfect home?

So I've found it very hard to make this leap. Because this enormous step—buying a house—is an incredible thing, an incredible opportunity . . . but it also shuts down so many other possibilities. We won't be moving to Italy anytime soon. And of course we were never going to—of course we weren't—but it was nice to think that maybe, just maybe, we might. We *could*. And if we make this decision . . . well, we can't. Not for a while, anyway.

But sometimes you need to just put on your Grown-up Pants and decide, already. Weigh the pros and cons, figure out what's important to you, argue with yourself to pieces . . . but then do it. Jump.

I have to say, though—I don't know that I would have had the courage to make that jump a year ago. But now it's not about us anymore, not really: It's about a little man who smiles so much when he looks out our New York City window, even when there's nothing to see outside but the apartment building across the way, that all we want to do is set him free to study the sky. And when we take that into account . . . well . . . it's not really a decision at all.

It's just what we're going to *do*.

And so we moved.

Out of the city, out of our sweet, slanty-floored little apartment, and into a brand-new life.

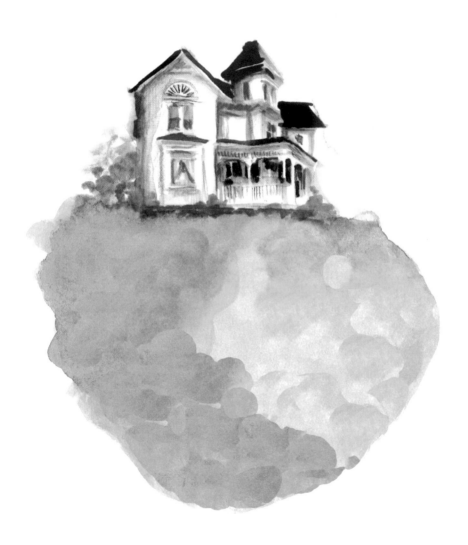

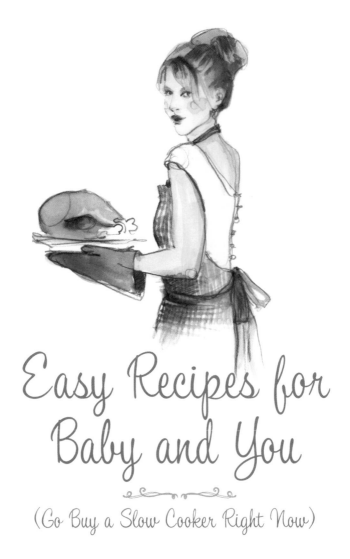

Easy Recipes for Baby and You

(Go Buy a Slow Cooker Right Now)

They Sell Those Fake Lemon Squeezy Bottle Things for a Reason, and That Reason Is "Babies"

When I told people that I was pregnant and nervous about the idea of bringing a baby home to a small walk-up apartment, the conversation—without fail—went something like this:

Me: "I'm nervous about bringing a baby home to a small walk-up apartment."

Unfailingly Positive Friend or Family Member: "Oh, it'll be great!"

Me: "I'll have to carry the stroller up and down four flights of stairs every time I leave the apartment."

UPFOFM: "No problem—you can get a light one!"

Me: "We have no closets."

UPFOFM: "Babies don't need much!"

Me: "The closest washing machine is four blocks away."

UPFOFM: "Just handwash the onesies and hang them on a line to dry! It'll be like you're Diane Lane in *Under the Tuscan Sun*, only in Manhattan and with a baby!"

Me: "We don't have a dishwasher."

Silence.

Me: "What?"

UPFOFM: "You should probably move."

Handwashing bottles, you see—each of which must first be broken down into eight thousand teeny-tiny individual parts, all of which may or may not have been glued to each other with cement—honestly just kind of sucks. Of course we did it, and it was fine, but let me tell you: when we first set foot in our new, dishwasher-including home, I literally got down on my hands and knees and hugged our appliance. (I really did. There's video evidence.)

The fact that we finally possessed not only a dishwasher, but also of a full-sized stove and an *actual countertop* meant that cooking became infinitely easier. But I have to tell you, working with the kinds of time and space constraints that we dealt with in those first few weeks and months with our son did wonders to help me abandon any precious ideas I had about dining and learn how to just get the food on the table, *now*.

Good food, of course. But easy food.

A caveat, before we go any further: If you are the type of person who cares about things like using exclusively fresh ingredients, chopping techniques, and whether your food once touched a non-organic atom or not . . . well, first, feel free to invite me over for dinner anytime. And second, this is probably not the chapter for you—go on and skip ahead to Chapter 6 so we can talk marital crises and postpartum depression; that'll be fun.

I mean, look, in a perfect world I'd mince up a bunch of fresh garlic cloves every time I was making a pasta sauce; of course I would, because fresh garlic is delicious. But in my life—my *real* life—the fact is that mincing garlic either makes my hands smell terrible for a bizarrely long time or requires me to clean out the fussy little garlic-mincer thing . . . and there's already a jar of garlic sitting right there in my refrigerator, looking all cute and pre-minced (I bought it in a weak moment, recalling how my mom always has a jar of garlic in her refrigerator and how truly awesome it is when I help her make dinner and do not have to mince garlic).

Besides, if anyone sitting down at my table were to ask me whether I had used fresh garlic they would (a) reveal themselves as an interloper (because I do not enjoy having friends who quiz me on things like whether I used fresh garlic), and (b) be lied to, because that's what you get when you ask such things of the person serving you dinner. I also may have used freshly squeezed lemons in that salad, or I may have just grabbed the fake lemon squeezy bottle thing sitting in my refrigerator door; I'm not telling.

Let's talk seriously fast food.

Pasta, Pasta, Pasta

They say that cooking with a newborn is a lost cause, but it's totally not. You just have to be flexible about both what you make and when you eat it. And whether or not it's warm and/or inhaled with the speed of a wild animal while precariously balancing a spoon over a very small, very adorable head.

What I've found helpful is to have a roster of meals at the ready that can be assembled in one (*maximum* two) pots, and that can be on the table in no more than half an hour. And for these purposes, there's nothing quite like a truly excellent pasta dish.

CRACK PASTA

I have such wonderful readers at Ramshackle Glam. They send me things like recipes for amazing pasta dishes, and I love them for it. This particular dish is based on a recipe emailed to me by a reader named Luisa years and years ago, and evolved over time into the version you see here. "Crack Pasta" is the name that Luisa bestowed upon it, and despite the changes I've made to the recipe over the years and the vague inappropriateness of including a reference to highly addictive narcotics in a book that's theoretically about new motherhood . . . it's a pretty apt descriptor. This pasta is addictive, and you will not be able to stop eating it. Don't say I didn't warn you.

SERVES 4–6

1 small yellow onion, finely chopped

6 to 8 slices lean bacon, cut into matchsticks

Extra-virgin olive oil

2 garlic cloves, minced

$3/4$ cup dry white wine

1 (28-ounce) can crushed tomatoes

Sea salt, to taste

Ground black pepper, to taste

1 box dried pasta of your choice

1 package steam-in-bag peas

$1/4$ cup heavy cream

Freshly grated Parmesan cheese (optional)

In a heavy-bottomed saucepan over medium heat, sauté the onion and bacon in a little olive oil until the bacon is cooked and the onions are translucent, adding the garlic halfway through.

Add the white wine to the saucepan and turn up the heat. Let the wine cook down a bit, until the smell of alcohol is more or less gone.

Add the tomatoes to the saucepan. Season to taste with salt and pepper, and give everything a good stir. Turn down the heat and let simmer for a few minutes (20 is ideal, but honestly, whatever).

Meanwhile, cook the pasta and steam the peas according to the package instructions.

Stir the heavy cream into the sauce and adjust the seasoning, if needed. Add the peas.

Strain the pasta (reserving a little pasta water) and toss it with the sauce, adding a little pasta water to loosen, if necessary. Top with Parmesan cheese, if desired.

NOTE: As with all the pasta dishes here, this recipe serves at least four people, and probably more. I like to make more than we'll eat in one sitting mostly because (1) I don't want to cook every night, and (2) I very much enjoy eating cold pasta for breakfast the next day (and think that you will, too).

MY KINDA BOLOGNESE

My mom made a version of this dish all the time when I was a kid, and it continues to be one of those meals that make me instantly happy. Especially if I'm watching The Waking Dead while eat– ing it, because tomato sauce and zombies make for a perfect storm of Things I Love.

SERVES 4–6

1 medium yellow onion, chopped

Extra-virgin olive oil

2 garlic cloves, minced

1 (28-ounce) can crushed tomatoes

Seasonings (options include red pepper flakes, summer savory, thyme, and rosemary . . . or nothing at all if you want to keep it easier-than-easy)

1 box pasta of your choice

1 package lean ground beef (approximately $^3/_4$ pound)

Sea salt, to taste

Ground black pepper, to taste

Place the onion and a little olive oil in a heavy-bottomed saucepan over medium heat. Cook, stir-ring occasionally, until the onion just begins to turn translucent. Add the garlic and cook for another minute or so, making sure that the garlic doesn't burn.

Add the crushed tomatoes and any other season-ings that you like, give the sauce a stir, and turn down the heat. Let the sauce simmer for about 20 minutes, stirring occasionally.

Meanwhile, bring a large pot of water to a boil and cook the pasta according to the package directions. When it's done, drain (reserving a little of the pasta water) and return it to the pot along with a splash of olive oil.

In a separate heavy-bottomed pan, cook the meat (breaking it up with the back of a wooden spoon) until it's cooked through (no longer pink).

Pour off the fat from the meat and add the meat to the tomato sauce. Continue simmering, adding salt and pepper to taste and adding a little pasta water to loosen, if necessary. Toss with the cooked pasta to serve.

CAPRESE PASTA

Caprese pasta (based on a recipe sent to me by a Ramshackle Glam reader named Felicity) is the best, especially in the summertime. Oh, and remember how I said in the Intro that I don't always care about using exclusively fresh ingredients? Well, I take it back for the moment: With this one I care, because when there are only four ingredients in a dish, they should probably all be pretty decent quality.

SERVES 4–6

1 package fresh pasta

1 ball fresh mozzarella

2 cups tomatoes, diced

1 large handful fresh basil, roughly chopped

All you do: Toss together the above ingredients in a bowl with some good extra-virgin olive oil and sea salt.

That's it.

Just One Fish Dish

The problem with fish is that babies don't seem to like it much, and neither does my husband. Which makes sense: I mean, it's fish. It can be fishy. Fish is also, however, quite delicious when done right (besides being *exceptionally* good for you), so I try to pull it into the roster at least once a week . . . and set aside a small portion for my son so that he can start acclimating those picky little taste buds.

One truly fantastic (and fantastically simple) fish dish will do for the time being.

SALMON WITH LEMON AND DILL

The best thing about this dish is that it's sort of impressive-looking even though it's pretty much the easiest thing ever, so it's a good one to call upon when you either have guests or want to make your significant other feel extremely guilty about the hours (hours!) you spent slaving over the stove. Bonus: cleanup involves...throwing out the foil. Done.

SERVES 2 . . .

with a little extra left over
for baby

2 teaspoons butter,
   cut into 2 pats

2 large salmon fillets

Extra-virgin olive oil

1 lemon (cut half into thin rounds;
   leave the other half intact to
   squeeze for juice)

$\frac{1}{3}$ cup dry white wine

1 small handful fresh dill, chopped

Sea salt, to taste

Ground black pepper, to taste

Green onions, chopped (optional)

Preheat the oven to 400°F.

Lay out a large square of aluminum foil (about 2$\frac{1}{2}$ feet should do the trick), and fold in half lengthwise. Fold up the sides of the foil to form a little box with an open top, and lightly butter the spot where you're going to place the salmon with half of the butter.

Set the salmon in the foil box, and drizzle with a little olive oil and squeeze the lemon half over the top. Pour in the white wine, then sprinkle with the chopped dill, along with a little salt and pepper.

Place the remaining pat of butter and a couple of the lemon slices in the foil box alongside the fish.

Close up the sides of the foil (make sure they're closed securely so the juice doesn't leak out) and bake for about 20 minutes, or until the fish flakes easily.

To serve, pour the sauce from the foil box over the fish, add a couple of the remaining lemon slices to each portion, and sprinkle with chopped green onions, if desired.

Serve alongside something green that makes you feel virtuous, like roasted asparagus or baby bok choy sautéed in olive oil and lemon.

MAKE IT EASIER!

Another nice thing about this dish is that it can be tweaked using whatever seasonings you have handy. Fresh lemon and dill are delicious and look really pretty, but if I've forgotten to stop into the market I'll just swap in a sprinkling of garlic powder or lemon pepper and call it a day.

The All-Stars

The two dishes here—one red meat, one chicken—are my all-stars: They're simple enough to whip up on a weekday (although the chicken needs to cook for a while, it's not labor-intensive at all), pretty enough to make for guests, and so, so good.

SKIRT STEAK & ARUGULA

Skirt steak is the best: It tastes amazing, it's cheap, and it's the fastest thing in the world to cook. You don't have to marinate the steak if you don't have time—a little salt will do—but if you can, you should. I never used to marinate meat; I sort of felt, you know: uggh, how annoying to have to (a) buy all those extra ingredients, (b) put in the extra time and effort to marinate, and (c) have to wash out a Ziploc afterward (I am a person who cannot throw away a Ziploc bag; it's weird). I thought that marinating couldn't really make that big of a difference, but as it turns out, marinating meat takes next to no effort at all, it's totally fun, and fills my improvisational inclinations nicely (you can just poke around in the refrigerator for things that sound like they might taste good on meat, and they probably will), and also? It makes a huge difference. Huge. Try it.

SERVES 4

BEST-EVER MARINADE

$1/2$ cup extra-virgin olive oil

$1/3$ cup soy sauce

3 minced garlic cloves, minced

1 tablespoon brown sugar

$1/2$ teaspoon Sriracha sauce

Sea salt, to taste

SKIRT STEAK & ARUGULA

1 pound skirt steak

4 to 6 cups arugula

$1/3$ cup extra-virgin olive oil

1 lemon

Combine all the marinade ingredients in a covered jar and shake well. Combine the steak and marinade in a large shallow dish or large zip-close plastic bag and marinate in the refrigerator for a minimum of 2 hours, then place on a very hot grill. This is going to cook fast—just 5 to 7 minutes on each side should do it.

Let the meat rest for about 10 minutes, and then slice into $1/2$-inch-wide slices, cutting across against the grain.

Toss the arugula in the olive oil and squeeze over the juice from the lemon. Season with salt and pepper, and arrange on plates with a few steak slices on top of each portion.

LEMONY ROAST CHICKEN

Roast chicken is one of those things that seem a little intimidating until you've actually done it, after which you discover that there's really nothing to it at all. You can make roast chicken as simple (just rubbed with olive oil and salt) or as complex (stuffed with everything from herbs to chopped prosciutto) as you want, but the one thing I insist on is that you separate the skin from the breasts and gently stuff a little softened butter into the space: The technique sort of self–bastes the chicken and adds a ton to the flavor.

SERVES 4–6

1 whole chicken
   (approximately 4 pounds)

Extra-virgin olive oil

Sea salt, to taste

1 lemon

2 garlic cloves, minced

$\frac{1}{2}$ stick unsalted butter,
   softened

Preheat the oven to 425°F.

Drizzle the chicken with olive oil and sprinkle it all over with salt.

With a vegetable peeler, remove a few strips of the bright yellow zest from the lemon, and finely chop (you want about a teaspoon's worth of chopped zest), setting the lemon aside for later.

Mash the chopped lemon zest and garlic into the softened butter.

Gently separate the skin covering the chicken's breasts from the meat, and use your fingers to push the butter mixture into the gap. Rub any remaining butter over the outside of the chicken.

Cut the lemon in half and push the two halves into the cavity of the chicken, leaving the flesh side of one half facing out for a pretty presentation.

Roast in the oven for about an hour and a half, or until an instant-read thermometer inserted into the thigh (not touching any bone) reads 165°F and the juices run clear.

Because Sometimes
You Want Something Green

I have this thing where I'm constantly saying I'm "not a salad person" . . . and it's true: I'm rarely thrilled to discover a pile of wilty green stuff sitting next to my hamburger in the spot where the French fries are supposed to go.

But I think I might totally be a salad person. Just a *picky* one. For me to want to eat a salad, you see, it must be something akin to spectacular. This salad? Spectacular.

CITRUSY CHICKEN & STRAWBERRY SALAD

SERVES 4

1 package chicken tenderloins (about 6 to 8 strips)

Garlic powder

Extra-virgin olive oil

$1/2$ lemon

1 large package mixed spring greens, washed and patted dry with paper towels

$1^1/2$ avocados, halved, pitted, peeled, and diced

$1/2$ cup fresh strawberries, sliced

$1/2$ cup sliced hearts of palm

Balsamic vinegar

Sea salt and ground black pepper, to taste

Cut the chicken tenderloins into chunks (about $1/2$ to 1 inch). Season with garlic powder.

Heat some olive oil in a heavy-bottomed skillet. Sauté the chicken until it is cooked through, adding the juice from the $1/2$ lemon toward the end of the cooking time. Remove to a plate to cool. When cool, cut chicken into smaller chunks (about $1/4$ inch).

In a large bowl, toss together the greens, chicken, avocados, strawberries, and hearts of palm with a little olive oil and balsamic vinegar. Season with salt and pepper to taste.

Go Buy a Slow Cooker Right Now

It is damn near impossible to cook anything fussy in close proximity to a toddler. I know this because whenever I try to make something even the tiniest bit complicated I end up sounding like this:

"Look, honey: Mommy's making dinner! You want to help? What a wonderful educational opportunity. Okay, first you put in the olive oil, and then . . . don't do that. Don't touch. No, you can't watch TV right now. Go play with—that's dog food, yuck yuck, don't touch. Okay, I can pick you up. Thank you for the hug. Can we hug after dinner is done? Thank you for the hug. Thank you for the hug. Okay, no more hugging. Thank you for the hug. That's a flower. Leaf. Flower. Flower. Flower. Don't touch. Mommy's dinner is burning, Mommy's putting you down now. No TV. Flower. Flower. Don't touch. Don't play with that, play with this. That's dog food, DON'T TOUCH."

. . . And that's when I turn on *Dora the Explorer*.

I'm not entirely certain how anyone put dinner on the table prior to the invention of Nick Jr., but it *had* to have involved a slow cooker. Honestly: Ten minutes of prep in the morning, and you return home at the end of the day to discover that your kitchen has gone ahead and cooked dinner for you.

Another reason I love slow cookers: They are totally unscrewupable. All you have to do is throw in some meat (cheap cuts are just fine; the slow-cooking will tenderize them), add a bunch of things that sound like they would taste good together, and then ignore it.

Presenting: two of my absolute favorite slow-cooker recipes.

SLOW COOKER POT ROAST

You know how people overuse the word "literally," and it's both incorrect and extremely annoying? "I literally flew over here!" "It literally scared me to death." "My dog literally just took apart my entire house." (Okay, I may have personally uttered that last sentence, and may indeed have meant it literally. But you understand what I'm saying.) This is literally the easiest one-pot meal in the world. Or at least in my world.

SERVES 4–6

Extra-virgin olive oil

1 boneless beef chuck roast
(about 2 pounds)

Season salt

Garlic powder

2 onions, peeled and quartered

1 (16-ounce) bag baby carrots

4 all-purpose potatoes, peeled
and cut into large chunks

Sea salt, to taste

Ground black pepper, to taste

Heat a few teaspoons of olive oil in a heavy-bottomed skillet or wide pot.

Generously season your roast with season salt and garlic powder, and then place in the pan, turning every couple of minutes so that it browns on all sides.

Put the vegetables in the slow cooker, and set the meat on top.

Turn the slow cooker to low, and leave it sitting there all day long, until the meat is fork tender (about 8 hours should do it). To serve, either slice the meat or shred it with a couple of forks, place in a bowl with the vegetables, and pour over the juices. Add salt and pepper, to season.

SLOW COOKER TURKEY CHILI

I've always been a bit wary of chili, because the few times I've had it it's been five-alarm spicy, and while a little heat is fine by me, I don't want my eating to involve pain. This chili, based on a hand-me-down recipe from my friend Anna, is painless. And flavorful. And inexpensive. And easy! All things I like.

SERVES 4–6

1¹/₂ to 2 pounds lean ground turkey

Garlic powder

Season salt

Extra-virgin olive oil

1 medium yellow onion, diced

1 green bell pepper, diced

1 (15-ounce) can black beans

1 (16-ounce) can tomato sauce

Half a packet of chili seasoning mix

Sea salt, to taste

Ground black pepper, to taste

TOPPING

Shredded cheese (I usually go for cheddar or a four-cheese mix)

Sour cream

Scallions, chopped

Very generously season the turkey with garlic powder and season salt. Add a little olive oil to a large pan and cook the turkey (breaking it up with the back of a wooden spoon) until it's cooked through, and no longer pink.

Remove the turkey meat to a slow cooker, and add all the remaining ingredients except for the topping ingredients.

Cook on high for an hour or two, then on low for another 7 hours or so. Check the seasoning every once in a while.

Serve with the toppings on the side.

When Your Inner Baker Calls

Sad, but true: If I were forced to bake in order to save my own life, I would probably end up dead. With cooking (or at least my kind of cooking), you get to just add a dollop here and a pinch there and things usually turn out more or less okay, but baking involves precision: one-eighteenth of a teaspoon of this and a thirtieth of an ounce of that and eight stirs per minute at a 45-degree angle and et cetera, et cetera.

I don't like doing it.

There is one thing, however, that I love to bake, and that I make whenever I'm feeling in need of something sweet that was not created in Mr. Hostess's factory (or when I am invited to someone's home for a meal and want to bring a respectably impressive contribution).

MOM'S BANANA BREAD

This banana bread recipe has been in my family for decades, and has never failed me. (Except for one time when I was in a rush and undercooked it and ended up with banana bread on the outside and banana soup on the inside. Don't do that.)

1 LOAF,
approximately 12 slices

¹/₂ cup softened butter

1 cup granulated sugar

2 eggs

2 cups all-purpose flour

1 teaspoon baking soda

¹/₂ teaspoon salt

3 very ripe bananas, mashed

¹/₂ cup Nutella (optional)

Preheat the oven to 350ºF.

Butter and flour a bread pan.

In a large bowl, cream the butter and sugar, then mix in the two eggs (one at a time).

In a separate bowl, sift together the flour, baking soda, and salt.

Gradually stir the sifted dry ingredients into the butter/sugar/eggs, and then mix in the mashed bananas.

Optional step: If you'd like to transform this into chocolate hazelnut banana bread, remove ¹/₂ cup of the batter from the bowl. Microwave the Nutella for a few seconds (not too much; you want it to soften but not burn), and stir it into the batter until well-blended. Fill the bread pan by alternating the regular batter and the Nutella batter, then lightly swirl with a knife.

Bake in the center of the oven for about an hour. (Make sure to test doneness with a toothpick, and note: Sometimes the hazelnut version can take a few minutes longer to cook.)

Homemade Baby Food

Oh, you didn't know that I make every single morsel that enters my son's mouth from scratch?

<Eye flutter.>

Please. I enjoy a nice overpriced prepackaged veggie blend as much as the next mama. But here's the thing: Once my son started eating more or less what we eat on a daily basis (just cut into smaller pieces), I realized that (a) we eat balanced meals *most* of the time, but certainly not *all* the time, and I'd really like our son to one-up us in the fresh-produce department, and (b) it's totally fun to cook for a small person who gets really excited by new tastes.

Oh yes, and it's cheaper.

You really can make an entire week's worth of veggie-blends with about forty-five minutes of time input per week, and it's so nice to be able to just reach into the freezer, pop out a cube or two, and have healthy options right there when you want them.

The possibilities for what you can make are endless, but what I do is this:

Add a sweetish fruit (like pear or apple) to a good-for-you vegetable that I wish was part of our family's "regular" diet but really isn't (like kale or broccoli).

Just boil, steam, or bake any fruits and vegetables that need to be softened, mash them together with a fork (or puree in a blender), add a little liquid (water, milk, or formula) to get the consistency you want, and season if desired. That's it. Really.

HOMEMADE BABY FOOD TIPS

• Buy seasonal produce; this saves you money and ensures that you're getting the freshest stuff available.

• Freeze your veggie blends in ice cube trays so that you can pop them out, defrost, and serve whenever you feel like your child's dinner could use a little boost.

• Switch up the texture based on your baby's age, making it chunkier (and thus more satisfying) as he or she gets older.

• Take advantage of leftovers: If you happen to make an extra-healthy veggie side dish for your family's dinner, just set a little aside, puree it, and put it in the freezer for later.

Important Note: What works for one baby doesn't necessarily work for all (especially when it comes to nutrition and the introduction of new foods), so please consult your pediatrician about any questions you may have.

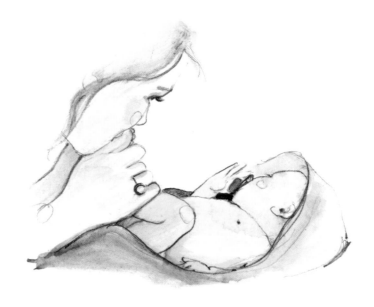

The Tough Stuff

(Let's All Screw Up Together)

A Peculiar Thing

Early on in my pregnancy, when I was busy tying myself up in knots about things like strollers and closets and finding room for bottle drying racks on our nonexistent countertop, one of the things I actually didn't worry a ton about, oddly enough, was . . . the baby. I just kind of figured he'd be okay. I mean, of course I went to all my doctor's appointments, ate decently, and avoided the stuff you're supposed to avoid, but mostly I just sort of got on with it and trusted that everything would turn out fine. He'd be born, and be loved and happy and ours, and our little family would roll on into wherever it was we were headed.

And then the strangest thing happened: A couple of months before my due date, my husband and I settled on a name for our son, and I started thinking about how I might want to share it on Ramshackle Glam. On my blog, you see, I share pretty much everything: career struggles; marital challenges; what eye cream I used last night; that time in seventh grade when I wore a brand-new outfit to school and then spilled a Snapple all over it and felt stupid . . . everything. I know lots of the people who read my site by their first names; they're my friends, and they're a real presence in my life—one that matters a lot. I'd already gone on and on (and on) about the fact that we were having a baby, and had even made a gender reveal video in which I cut into a blue cake while wearing way too much jewelry and sort of shrieking and hopping around. I had been writing about imminent motherhood for months, and talking about the process of selecting a name for our child felt like a natural part of that.

So I sat down, started typing out a "We Picked a Name!" post, and that's when the strange thing happened:

I panicked.

I use the word panic a lot because . . . well, I panic a lot, I guess, but this time I mean *panicked*, italics and intense physical reaction and all: I got flushed and dizzy, my heart started ping-ponging around in my chest, and I thought, "You know what? Let's move my seven-months-pregnant self away from the computer and chill out for a second."

So that's what I did. I figured sooner or later I'd work out whatever was putting me into such a state, but in the meantime I'd just keep on referring to our unborn son as "Indy"—the pseudonym we'd picked out a few months earlier, when we still hadn't been sure what we were going to call our child.

But I didn't work out why even the thought of sharing my son's name made me so upset. Not for a long time.

On the morning that our son came into the world, I put up a "He's here!" photo on my Facebook page accompanied by his first name, went back to my bed to lie down . . . and boom, it happened again: the panic thing. I shot up out of a dead sleep and raced (or, more accurately, shuffled) over to my computer and edited the caption out of the post, hoping that I'd moved quickly enough that nobody had seen it. For whatever reason deleting his name made me feel better, and back to sleep I went.

Now, people's feelings about social media and sharing certainly run the gamut, and it's definitely not out-of-the-ordinary (or without reason) for a new parent to think twice about sharing any information whatsoever about their child in a public forum, be it Twitter, Facebook, a blog, or any other outlet that can be viewed by more than the most immediate friends and family . . . but the fact is that my anxiety was very much out-of-character for me. I'm a person who sifts through my life as source material as a matter of course, both because I enjoy the process and because it's simply how I operate. I genuinely believe in the value of sharing personal experiences with others, and being open even with people I don't know is something that I am nearly always comfortable with. Beyond that, my husband and I had revisited the idea of having me explore the experience of parenthood in my writing time and again, and had jointly decided that we were secure in this decision.

Given all this, the amount of distress I was feeling about sharing my son's name—such a small thing, in the scheme of the things that I share—seemed . . . if not "unfounded," at the very least "peculiar."

Peculiar, that is, until much later on, when I finally understood what was going on in my head, and what was going on was this: Something about sharing my son's name made him real. He wasn't going to stay safely tucked away forever; he was going to be here, a person in the world, and a person who the world could hurt in ways that I wouldn't necessarily be able to see coming.

In the years since my son has arrived I have posted countless photos and videos that include my family, and yet I continue to use a pseudonym for my son on my website. And although of course my husband and I are entitled to make whatever decisions we feel are appropriate for our family, I understand why this may be a confusing choice . . . mostly because it's one that I've had a great deal of trouble understanding myself. So let me explain.

For my generation at least, the Internet can sometimes feel like the place where your story is written. And while I write every day about my life and about my experiences as a mother, I do not want to write my son's story for him.

I am a person who has made certain choices, for better or for worse, and one of those choices was to make my life—and to some extent my family's life—something that is out there for people who want to read about it to see, debate, even judge, but still: My son's tale—the goings-on of his mind and heart and self—is his to reveal if and how he sees fit. The truth is that I do sometimes question my choice to share my family—of course I do—and so I want to take care that this single small thing, this silly matter of a website, doesn't pepper itself too densely over a world that my son will one day claim for himself, in his own way.

I tell stories about my son because the space that he consumes in my mind and my heart is too big for me to secret away; for me, to write without writing of my child would be to dance circles around the truth. But who I see, who I write about . . . that is a different person than who he is. It can be difficult for a person—for everyone—to remember that what people say about you and who you are is not one and the same, and so it was important to me that I not write my son's name hundreds, perhaps thousands of times in a public space before he has the opportunity to learn how to form those letters himself.

In the beginning, of course, my choice (if you could even call it that) wasn't this reasoned. And it wasn't even about a name. It was about my desire to wrap my son up in my arms and run with him far away to where no one could ever make him cry.

I wanted to control it all, you see. Everything.

I didn't know how I would handle all the bad things in the world that might harm my baby boy, and so I gathered them up into this one small fear: the fear that someone on the Internet might say something mean about my child, and that he might one day search for his name and read that mean thing and be hurt by it. I couldn't take the idea of him being hurt at all. Ever. I wanted to hide him from all the things in the world that I feared would harm him beyond repair and turn him inward, to a place where I wouldn't be able to reach him anymore.

What I was scared of more than anything were the wounds that I might not be able to see, and so I picked one that I could.

My son is barely into toddlerhood now, and the things that hurt him are a skinned knee, or a dog that's licked him too enthusiastically, or a toy that's been taken away. These are small injuries, and they are ones that I can see right in front of me, that I can at least try to shield him from. I can kiss a cut, push away a dog, explain why sharing is often better than having. But I know that there are days right around the corner when my son will come home from school in tears over someone's words, something he heard or read or suspected was said. The chances are excellent that people are going to say mean things to him, about him. Of course they are, because this is the kind of thing that happens. To everyone. Because their parent has a website; because of a picture posted on Facebook; because of a rumor, a whisper, a grudge; because of none or all of these things. And my job is not to pretend that such things do not happen, but to help him learn how to handle them if—when—they do.

I made a choice early on in parenthood that was a reaction to fear, not a thoughtful decision. Even so, it's one that I continue to maintain, albeit for a different reason. Not because my son's name is a secret—it's not, it's right there in the acknowledgments in the back of this book, where I thank him alongside many of the other people I love most in the world—but rather to remind him that his mother may write of him, but she does not tell his story.

And neither does anyone else, no matter how many words they may use.

I want my son to know that he can exist right alongside the enormous variety of opinions in this world, all those beliefs and ideas and thoughts that run from the thoughtful and kind all the way to the illogical and terrifying. More than that, I want him to know that he can hear all these thoughts, let them in, open himself up even to conflict and differences and sadness and anger . . . and still decide for himself what path he will take. I want him to know that those voices that can hurt are out there, but that his voice is louder. And most of all, I want to teach him to look his fears straight in the eye, figure out for himself what is true and what is not, and then climb right on over all those countless things that people may say, leaving their words way back there in the dust and the weeds, where they belong.

In the Deep

My struggles with anxiety started when I was fourteen years old and I couldn't figure out how to become a grown-up while still getting to hang out in the cheerful semi-obliviousness of childhood. I remember in elementary school overhearing a friend say that her father was "depressed" and thinking, "Well, that's weird. Why would anyone ever be depressed when there's so much to be happy about in the world?"

Sweet, right?

And then, as I made my way into early adulthood and started to feel the possibilities for what could happen to me and to the people I loved widen every day, the edges of all that happiness began to curl up a little bit, and fear came creeping in along with the future.

Over the years my episodes have come and gone, moving in and out of my life in almost negligible relation to actual circumstances, but really: Anxiety has skittered around in the periphery of my mind for long enough that you'd think it might have at least occurred to me that experiencing some degree of postpartum emotional upheaval would be a real possibility.

Nope.

I had heard of postpartum depression and the "baby blues," of course, and knew because I am not a Bot that lots of people suffer from these conditions and that they're not actually things that anyone *chooses* to have, but still: Deep down, I thought that there was no way it could possibly happen to me. I mean, how could I feel sad with an adorable little baby sitting right there next to me?! That would be crazy!

Call me crazy.

When we were getting ready to leave the hospital, I laid my two day-old son down on the bed to button up his tiny onesie, and was suddenly absolutely crushed—I mean *crushed into pieces*—by how frail he looked lying there on that mattress, practically swimming in the outfit that I'd chosen for his big day even though it was the smallest one we owned. I cried while tucking him into his car seat, then cried my way through the hospital lobby, then cried all the way back to our apartment with our very nervous taxi driver, and then couldn't stop crying and didn't know what to do about it.

I didn't even know *why* I was crying; not exactly. Sure, there were some actual, concrete fears floating around in my head, but most of it was a big old ball of Does Not Compute, and when what you're sad about are things that you can't even begin to geolocate in your head—forget about putting them into actual *words*—it's pretty difficult to talk yourself out of them.

The pain didn't make any logical sense to me, but it was still so overwhelming that it made me do something that I really do not like to do: I turned to my husband and told him that I could not continue feeling this way, and that I needed help. I don't know that I've ever said those words so plainly in my life, or meant them so much.

"I need help," I said . . . and I did, I really did. And he saw that I was telling him the truth, and promised me that we would get me that help. The next morning we went to the doctor, where I was given a prescription that took the sharpest edges off of what I was feeling and left me able to smile at the baby who was curling his tiny fingers around my own, looking for something to hold on to in his brand-new world. I hated that I needed a pill to help me handle those first few weeks . . . but I did.

I really did.

And you know what? That's just fine.

"Ask for help when you need it." Big deal, right? But it's one thing to "know" it—and another thing to *do* it. Because when you need help, absolutely *require* it if one foot is going to keep going in front of the other, it's scary. When that need then coincides with a moment you've been frightened you wouldn't live up to in the first place—a moment when you are suddenly responsible for an entire other human being's *existence* and want nothing more than to be not just competent, but *perfect* in this pursuit—that just makes it all the harder to admit you can't go it alone.

What I know now: There is enormous strength in being able to admit that you need help, and in then being willing to ask for it. Sometimes you have to fight for your health, for your happiness, for your peace . . . and the very bravest thing you can do is reach out for a hand to hold on to while you take your next steps, whatever they may be.

It's the steps themselves that are the important part, not whether or not you go them alone.

"BABY BLUES" . . . OR POSTPARTUM DEPRESSION?

Over 50 percent of women suffer from baby blues just after childbirth. The symptoms include mood swings, weepiness, stress, anxiety, and forgetfulness. They typically disappear within two weeks following childbirth, once hormonal changes have settled down.

If the blues continue for more than two weeks after childbirth, the condition is now considered PPD. Symptoms can include a combination of any of the following: depressed mood, loss of pleasure, appetite changes, fatigue, guilt, hopelessness, or helplessness, attention/concentration troubles, indecisiveness, and thoughts of suicide or homicide.

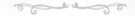

WHEN TO ASK FOR HELP

If your baby blues persist for more than two weeks, you should seek help as you have likely developed PPD. If at any point (even sooner than two weeks postpartum) you find that you are unable to function and suffer from strong depression, guilt, anger, appetite loss, or suicidal or homicidal thoughts, it is imperative that you seek help immediately. Effective treatment is available for PPD, and early intervention is key to getting you on track and helping you to enjoy time with your baby.

*Source: Shelby Harris, PsyD, licensed Clinical Psychologist and Assistant Professor of Neurology and Psychiatry at the Albert Einstein College of Medicine.

Baby Insecurity and Why You're Just Fine

There is not a day that goes by when I'm not at least a little bit grateful that my son isn't so hot in the Memory Department yet. Let's be honest: It is a virtual guarantee that over the course of any given twenty-four hour period I will do something that I do not want my child to remember and/or repeat, whether that's slamming a door, arguing with my husband, giving up and just making macaroni and cheese for dinner (the neon kind, not the fancy kind), or calling my dog a not-so-nice name because of what he just did to my carpet.

Let me take you back to when my son was five months old and sitting on my lap in the nursery, enjoying some nice, secure, two-handed support from a mother whose attention was completely and fully on him. I'm serious: I was not only looking directly at him, thinking about him, and probably cherishing him . . . I was *physically touching him with every single one of my limbs.* Half a second later he was facedown on the floor, having somehow done a tiny surprise jig that catapulted him off of my lap and onto the rug. I continue to have no idea how this happened, but it made me (and presumably my child) feel terrible.

When he was eight months old, my son started practicing his "pull up" technique anywhere and everywhere he could, especially in extremely unsafe places where I would have really preferred he didn't. In the apartment where we lived during much of his first year our bathroom didn't have enough floor space to fit the baby bathtub, so we had to sort of prop it sideways in the hallway. During one of those baths when he decided to do water gymnastics I started trying to maneuver him back down into a more bathing-appropriate position . . . and my hands slipped on his soapy little body. And he went shooting out of the bathtub and sliding down the length of our hallway on his belly, eventually coming to rest at the entrance to our living room: slightly stunned, possibly a little annoyed at me, but basically fine.

When he was eleven months old, I managed to lock him in my car . . . or, rather—just to offload a tiny bit of the blame, here—*he* locked *himself* in the car. Because I had given him the keys to play with. And in the two-second interlude between when I closed the back door and went to open the front door, he managed to hit the "GIVE MOM A HEART ATTACK BY LOCKING HER OUT" button, and then reacted to my frantic efforts to magically transform him into an older person (one capable of understanding instructions like "Please hit the unlock button") by smiling and hurling the keys into the trunk. Fact: You have never seen anyone sing "The Wheels on the Bus" with their face smashed against a car window as cheerily or as loudly as I did for the fifteen minutes that it took to get that door open.

So that was a fun little episode. It even resulted in the opportunity to make some brand-new friends: the police officers in charge of protecting our town from people who lock their children in cars.

Then, about a week after we moved into our new house, I learned that the door leading out to our porch locks automatically when it closes. Unfortunately, I learned this while standing on the "outside" side of the door, holding a one-year-old.

Let's go ahead and lay this one out:

1. Blonde girl;
2. Holding cute baby;
3. Wearing next-to-nothing (whatever, it was seventy zillion degrees and I was cleaning);
4. Standing alone on a very small, very high-up patio in a quiet, suburban neighborhood;
5. Literally screaming at the top of her lungs for help.

I continue to be surprised that the next thing that happened wasn't that the Loch Ness Monster rose up out of the lake, made his way over to our house and ate me, because that is what usually happens next in that kind of movie. What *actually* happened was that a man heard me screaming, came walking out of the woods, very fortunately turned out to be my next-door neighbor rather than a serial killer, and freed us from our little predicament.

Anyway, you screw up a lot when you have kids. Or maybe it's that you screw up a lot generally (or at least I do), but when you have kids you just *notice* it more, because you do something screwed-up and instantly realize, Oh. I totally just screwed up my child.

Having children is like a crash course in All the Ways You Do Stuff Wrong, and that nowadays includes not only stuff that makes logical parenting sense (like, say, not allowing your dogs to babysit or feeding your child a steady diet of Ho Hos), but also stuff like using "teaching language." As an example, apparently you're supposed to tell you child not that he is "good" or "bad," but that he displays "good or bad *behaviors*" so that he doesn't think that the relative goodness or badness of his actions speaks to the relative goodness or badness of *him*. This makes total sense in theory; in practice, it makes me crazy.

What's especially fun is when you top all these things that you feel like you're doing wrong with a big old case of Mommy Brain—which, just so you know, is a real thing. There was one day, I (sort of) remember, when I spent a full half hour hunting around our apartment for our stroller, only to discover that I'd apparently walked down four flights of stairs, deposited it in the foyer of our apartment building, and then walked back up all four flights . . . with zero recollection of the entire trip. I followed up this odd little incident by going into the kitchen to unpack the many bags of groceries that I'd just lugged upstairs, being unable to find them *anywhere* . . . and then discovering that I'd already put them away. All of them.

And I could not remember doing it.

I'm sorry, but that is *weird*. And sort of stressful, the whole idea of not necessarily being able to rely on your brain to function appropriately during a time when you especially wish it would.

You know what else can really stress a mom out? Other moms. I don't know how it happened that all of the mothers in the world turned out to be perfect, but that's what it seems like according to the Internet. That's also what it seems like on my local playground: Every single other mom hanging around the jungle gym always seems to have a battalion of sunscreen, extra diapers, tissues, educationally sound toys, and organic snacks at the ready, and over there in the corner is me, flailing around in my purse in search of anything—seriously, *anything*—that will double as a tissue before giving up and sacrificing the sleeve of my shirt to the Nose Gods.

But it's true, you know: Even those moms on the playground who look—from the outside, at least—like they have it all together . . . they have those moments, too. Lots of them.

Everyone feels like they're a terrible parent sometimes. Everyone has those days when they mess up, or do something they wish that they hadn't, or just don't feel like they can be the one in charge for one single more second. Some days your child will simply not stop crying for no good reason at all, and it can feel like he is miserable and will always *be* miserable, and you have failed at the one thing that you want the most: to make your baby happy.

In this week's issue of my *Star* magazine there is an article on "grading" celebrity moms. Nicole Richie gets a C, because she admitted that she sometimes thinks it's funny when her son falls.

Let's be real clear on this point: It *is* sometimes funny when children fall. (Not when they're *hurt*, when they *fall*. That's an important distinction.)

Other celebrities got "bad grades" for everything from co-sleeping to leaving their children with others while they go to work to throwing extravagant birthday parties: all actions that are not only hugely subjective, but are also just a small fraction of the enormous spectrum of things that make up who one is as a parent. The article was meant to be silly, I'm sure, but I can't help but think that it's damaging, the perpetuation of this idea that mothers are "good" or "bad" based on their individual choices and parenting styles. Being a great parent isn't about remembering to bring tissues with you every time you go to the playground, or whether you buy the organic apple-sauce, or whether you child uses a pacifier for a few months beyond when his best friend does. The possibilities that parenthood can bring are almost infinite, and what works for one mother and one family may not work at all for another.

It's not confined to celebrities, of course. All this is just an amped-up version of what's going on with regular old non-celebrity mothers every single day. I've personally been stopped on the street by total strangers and lectured about everything from the presence or absence of my son's socks to the exact degree to which his blanket should be tucked in around him to the length of his hair and whether or not it's appropriate for a boy (this last guy barely escaped without his McDonald's milkshake getting upended on his head). Judgment is everywhere, and it is loud, and it can be very scary to admit that you feel like you're not completely perfect at the one job in the world that you want to be perfect at more than any other.

From time to time I get emails from young women who want to pursue a career in writing and ask if I have any advice to help them find their "voice." And what I tell them, every time, is this: just write. A lot. Because if you're putting your words into the world every single day, as much as you can, your voice just comes out; you can't stop it. It'd be too exhausting to be disingenuous that much.

In some ways, I've experienced something similar with motherhood. When I thought about parenting before I ever became a parent, I figured I'd approach motherhood the way I've approached most things in my life: by consciously evaluating the pros and cons, deciding on the best course of action, and then doing just that. Well, maybe you could parent in exactly the way you'd like to for an afternoon . . . but for years? Decades? Whether you try to micro-manage every minute or just let things be, you can't help it . . . who you are, deep-down, just *comes out*. And if your face lights up the way that I am certain that it does when you look at your child, that is what is going to rise above all that other noise, those mistakes and imperfections and screw-ups. Your voice. Your voice saying "I love you" and meaning it more than you've ever meant anything in your life.

TIME-SAVERS THAT (REALLY) WORK

One of the major things that can leave you feeling overwhelmed is the too-much-to-do/too-little-time thing. I get it. I have too much to do and not enough time, also. These easy little fixes help a *ton*:

PUT BABY TO BED. I completely understand the impulse to let your child stay up a little later from time to time. "Oooh!" you think, "I'll get an extra hour of sleep!" No. You won't. Bizarrely enough, the reverse is true: putting children to bed earlier makes them sleep better and longer, and when children sleep better and longer it's all kinds of wonderful.

DO SOME NIGHTTIME PREP TIME. Once my son goes to sleep I want nothing more than to turn into a statue in front of the TV, but I do not. Instead, I transform into a little multitasking hero. I prep his lunch, straighten up the kitchen so that I don't have to wake up to a disaster zone, and go over my to-do list for the next day, checking off anything small that I can take care of in advance.

PICK YOUR BATTLES. One thing I do *not* do the night before is lay out my son's clothing—because pulling a T-shirt and a pair of jeans out of a drawer is not exactly rocket science—but if I had a little girl and had the yen to put her in things like hair bows and tights and outfits that match? I'd totally do the night-before clothing lay-out. Your call.

SAY NO TO NEAT DRAWERS. Just throw all those bed sheets right on in there. A wrinkle or two won't kill anyone, folding next to a toddler who thinks a pile of fresh laundry is a Magical Mystery House is an exercise in futility, and honestly: Who cares?

MAKE EVERY TRIP COUNT. My #1 keep-your-house-neat tip: every time I walk through my house—and I mean *every single time*—I pick something up and return it to its rightful place. Socks under the table? Straight into the laundry basket. Random Matchbox car? Dropped off in the toy box on my next pass by. Errant receipt? Into the receipts file (or the trash, depending on how responsible I'm feeling) it goes. This keeps things more or less in order, so I almost never have to do big picking-up sessions. (Except for when it comes to Legos, which apparently multiply like little Mogwais and enjoy finding hiding places in every single corner of our home.)

BECOME A LIST WIZARD. If you make lists for everything, you don't have to remember anything. This is fantastic. It's also especially helpful for groceries: I keep an ongoing list in my phone of the stuff we've run out of so that I don't have to waste time peeking through my cabinets before every trip to the store.

MAKE A MEAL PLAN. Speaking of groceries, I put together a (very rudi-mentary) meal plan at the beginning of each week so that I can get the major-ity of my shopping done in one trip. Sure, I have to make the occasional quick stop for something I've forgotten, but a quick stop is way better than a full-on stroll through the aisles with a small person who needs to touch every. single. banana.

BE BUSY. The very best way to extend a nap: Make sure you have some-where that you really, really have to be. Make plans for the time that your child typically wakes up, and make sure that they're extremely important. Your child will sleep forever and ever and ever.

Pressure Times Two

You know how when you're single, all anyone wants to know is if you're dating anyone? And then the second you start getting serious with someone, the only question people have for you is "When are you getting engaged?" And then: "When are you getting married?" and "When are you having kids?" And it's super-annoying, because you wish that people would just let you exist in the moment that you're in for a minute before rushing you into whatever's next?

It doesn't stop there. The second—and I mean the *second*—you actually give birth, all anyone wants to talk about are the two following topics:

1. How fast it all goes and how desperately sad you'll be when your children are grown;

2. When you're going to have another.

And if you answer "We're not" or even "I don't know" to the second question, you better be ready to explain yourself. I understand that there is no malicious intent here, only a desire to help and guide . . . but still: It's absolutely zero fun to be stopped on the street by a total stranger who touches your child's feet with a wistful expression and tells you that he'll be gone before you know it, and that you better hurry up if you want to have more children (who will then grow far too fast in their own turn). I am sure that people who do this are trying to be nice. It's horribly upsetting.

I am so aware—*so aware*—that every day that passes is a day with my son that I will never have again. The constant reminders of "how fast it goes" and that I "have to savor every minute"? You know what they're doing? They're making me so freaked out about all this savoring that I'm getting pulled right out of where I'm trying to be; every second, I'm thinking "Am I enjoying this *enough*?"

Sometimes I sit in the nursery with my son and watch him play, and honestly? I really want to pick up an *US Weekly* and read about Christina Aguilera while he does his thing . . . but I can't. Because I am so terrified of turning around, and in the blink of an eye he'll be grown and out the door, and I'll spend every day for the rest of my life wishing I had chosen to watch him roll his ball for that one moment rather than do something—anything—else.

This is, of course, irrational. But it's also impossible to get away from, and the sheer volume and repetition of "your children will grow up far too fast" is enough to break anyone's heart.

Sometime around my son's first birthday, I started realizing that as long as that first year had taken, it was over now, and the realization sent me reeling. I was excited to see where my son was headed, but devastated by the fact that moving on meant leaving some things behind.

I didn't want my baby's babyhood to go. It was too wonderful. And as the turn of his first year approached, the noise all around me, the noise in my head—"When's the next one? When when when?"—grew louder.

Savor The Moment (That's an Order)

Do we want to have another child? I think so. I don't know. I know that I did wish that I had a sibling growing up, and I wish I had one even now. I also know that I got to do extremely cool things with my parents that I may not have gotten to do had there been another child around. I know that if we only have one child, he'll have a very different kind of life—more exciting and easier in some ways, less exciting and harder in others—than if we give him a brother or sister. I know that if we do decide to have another we'll love him or her madly and won't be able to imagine our lives any other way.

I also know that having a child is in many ways a stroke of the best luck you can ever have, and it may not even be up to us to decide. And whatever ends up happening, of course it's nobody's business but our own, but that's not what's at stake here. I'm not worried that other people will think we made the wrong decision; I'm worried that if we wait too long or decide not to have another baby for whatever reason, that one day I'll think that *I* did.

Most of all, I'm worried that I'll spend the time that I get with my son—this precious time in the months and years after he first arrived in this world—so focused on the future and our plans and what could be that I'll forget to pay attention to what *is*.

Being brave and taking the leap is important—I believe that—but sometimes staying exactly where you are for a moment is just what you need in order to decide how to move forward . . . or if you're going to at all.

Sometimes the "right here, right now" isn't a place you're in a rush to leave.

Oh, Right ... I'm Married

I threw a remote control at my husband the other night.

Why?

Because he forgot to set the DVR to tape *The Bachelorette*. And then he tried to fix it, and in the course of his efforts ended up turning off the part of the television that refuses to reboot without the assistance of a platoon of Navy SEALS, which resulted in me missing the live version as well.

And I'll tell you what: Every single Mom Friend of mine who I've told this story to has responded with, "That makes sense." *The Bachelorette* is crucial stuff.

I'm kidding, of course. (Not about the actual throwing; that happened. Don't throw remotes at your husband.)

It's just a fact: Having a child throws some pretty intense wrenches into your relationship. Some of the ways that it changes things are wonderful: Having a baby puts all those minor disagreements into perspective (with a possible exception for truly excellent reality TV shows that have not been recorded when someone *promised me that they were*) and makes you more interested in communicating your way through disagreements than yelling. It forces you to see what you're fighting about through young (and impressionable) eyes, and you finally (finally!) understand that the most important thing is not "winning," but rather arriving at a solution that works for everyone.

It makes you realize that you're in it—all of it—together.

But a marriage—especially one in the midst of a massive transition—can't be all smiles and fabulous learning opportunities. Bringing a child into the mix can also make your relationship a lot more challenging, mostly because enormous life transformations that require you to confront your most deeply seated beliefs—and then find a way to blend them with the most deeply seated beliefs of an entirely separate person who presumably comes to the table with his or her own set of ideas about how things should and should not be done—have the tendency to do that.

Also: Adapting to an entirely new way of living on very little sleep is just really freaking difficult.

I used to have actual, full-sentence-inclusive conversations with my husband, you know. But for the first few months after our son arrived, my daily communications with Kendrick were all via text message, and all went something like this:

Him: "Want me to bring anything home for you?"

Me: "Obi it."

Him: "What?"

Me: "Hohoho."

Autocorrect is not a friend of those who must type with one hand while holding a baby with the other.

It's an understatement to say that in the very beginning things were tough with us. Not bad, exactly, just . . . different, and different in a way that made me a little sad. We were just so *serious* so much of the time, so wrapped up in and focused on how to handle this new responsibility, and we bore very little resemblance to the fantasy I had in my head of lighthearted, blissed-out parents who walked around all drunk on joy and wonder over what they'd created 24/7.

When I was pregnant, I made a promise to myself to continue to prioritize our relationship even after the baby arrived. I genuinely internalized how important this was to me, but even though I truly believed that the very best thing that we could do for our son was to have a happy, healthy marriage . . . I couldn't do it. For a little while right in the beginning, I couldn't even *see* my husband; all I saw was our son, and what needed to be done for him, and if everything was fine with him, there were a million other things that needed to be taken care of before I could turn my attention to my marriage. Or rather a million and one, because once my son went down for a nap what was going to happen before anything else was that I was going to ingest my 500-ounce Red Bull, because that was what gave me the energy to check my email or to speak.

Sure, I kept going through the motions of things that I believed would keep my marriage strong—making rudimentary attempts at actual adult conversation, finding time for the occasional Date Night—but it felt like I had blinders on, and my husband was on the other side of those blinders, and pretty much anything he said or did that wasn't directly helping me handle all the things I had to do made me *nuts*. I honestly just didn't really care about how his day had gone, and that's something that I was used to caring about very much. We were often too tired to fight, but when we did the speed with which those arguments escalated scared me. I was stunned by how easily the emotional hailstorm of new parenthood could overwhelm our ability to treat each other the way we wanted to, the way we had grown used to and expected. I started feeling competitive about who was working harder; who had the tougher day-to-day schedule. *Me*, I thought. OBVIOUSLY. It felt like it was all just too much.

It was. Too much. That was it: why I didn't really care about how his day had gone; why I sometimes got so overwhelmed that my frustration emerged as anger; why I threw that remote. From time to time all that responsibility, all those musts and have-tos and right-nows that come along with adulthood can feel like way more than a single person—or even a pair of people—can handle, especially when it's all very new and you haven't yet found the tools that work for you.

Nobody wants to fight with the person they married. Nobody wants to raise their child in a house filled with screaming and tears rather than patience and compassion. But the reality is that people sometimes get overwhelmed, and sometimes respond to conflict in a way that they wish they hadn't. In a way that they wish they could take back.

You know what the number-one most valuable thing that having a baby has taught us?

To let each other *take it back*.

It is so important to be thoughtful about your relationship, and to approach it with care and attention . . . but it's also important to remember that it's okay to be less than the most perfect version of yourself once in a while, when things get really crazy. When your life undergoes a dramatic change—and the introduction of a brand-new family member is an enormous change, no matter who you are or what your lifestyle was like prior to the baby's arrival—things can get weird, and it can help to acknowledge that weirdness and make the conscious choice to not sound the alarms. To hold off on making grand statements about the future of your marriage or how Things Are Different, and to let yourself be tossed around a little and have faith that when the waters settle down, there you'll both be.

There are many things—oh, so many things—that I wish I could do better. I wish I didn't feel like I need to prove to my husband that my day was more difficult than his; I wish that I didn't shut down when what I need to do is open up; I wish that I was able to take off the blinders more often and see that he needs something, and what that something is, is *me*. I wish I could do better, *be* better, but I think that the wishing is the part that really matters: the desire to keep moving forward, and to keep moving forward *together*.

All that time that we've spent learning about each other, both before and after our son's arrival, you see: It's created a foundation. One that has built up over time, and one that will hopefully let us bend a little when we need to.

Couples fight; that's just the way it goes. But once in a while, you have to let each other take it back.

And then let it go.

How-To: RECONNECT FOR A SEC

Some days—or weeks—you're just not going to feel like adding "remembering that my partner is a human being, too" to the list of things that you have to accomplish. One thing that I have discovered, though, is that every single time—and I mean *without fail*—that we put even the tiniest bit of extra effort into reconnecting, we're happy we did. It's *always* worth it.

LAUGH IT OUT. One of my favorite things that having a baby has done to our relationship is that it has rendered about 85 percent of the fights that we have completely ridiculous. We'll be mid-yell about something or other, and then all of the sudden one or both of us will realize that what we're yelling about is whether or not the little trap in the kitchen sink has been emptied and whose fault it is . . . and we will start cracking up. This is great. There are bigger things to worry about—bigger things that are sure to create their own conflicts from time to time, too—and it can help a ton to let the small stuff slide.

GO AWAY. Sometimes you need to just get out and go anywhere. A week-end at a resort is lovely, but the coffee shop down the block will do just fine; the important thing is that the two of you are physically together and also physically separated from all the things (jobs, chores, even—yes—children) that can sometimes make you nuts.

PUT IT ON PAUSE. I'm one of those people who straightens up before heading to bed every single night; I just don't like waking up to things like pil-lows all over the floor or a sink full of dishes. Once in awhile, though, I manage to shut off that part of my brain and let everything on our list go for the night so we can just settle in with a movie and each other. Sometimes the other stuff can wait.

STAY SAFE. Having a "safety word" (a nonsense word or phrase that either of you can use as a virtual "Pause" button during an argument) may feel ludi-crous . . . but it's kind of the best. One of the most effective ways to reconnect is to avoid getting really nasty in the first place, and "safety words" can help put a disagreement on ice for the time being so that you can both take a few deep breaths that may keep you from saying something you don't mean. (Incidentally, it also helps if your safety word is something guaranteed to make you both laugh, because it's very difficult to argue with someone who is screaming "DEBBIE GIBSON" at you. For example.)

Wild Nights and Where I Went

I'm not anywhere near as "fun" as I used to be.

I'm using the word *fun* in the very most clichéd of ways, of course—the way that a teenager would use the word. ("*God*, mom, you're *no fun*." Like that.)

What I mean is really that the "old me" was . . . a little wild. Spontaneous to a fault. Even—yes—stupid on occasion, and way too interested in risk-taking for my own good. (Sometimes I think about my twenty-three-year-old self and just want to scoop her up and drop her in the middle of Montana for a couple of years, so she can get whatever was in her system out in relative safety.)

These days, I'm just not anything even approximating "wild"; you're not going to find me out past midnight . . . ever, really. A few weeks ago, our friends came over for an afternoon BBQ and ended up staying until around 11:30 p.m., at which point I more or less threw them in the direction of the train station. I mean, I am *tired*. And I wake up at six, because that's when the sun gets up, and our son really enjoys getting up with it.

I was telling some of my "back in the L.A. days" stories to a new friend at a party the other weekend, and she said, "Wow, we should go to Vegas together sometime. It sounds like you'd be a lot of fun." Nope. If you took me to Vegas, I'd probably plant myself in a spa, eat sushi until it came out my eyeballs, and then pass out for twelve hours. I mean, *I* think that sounds fun . . . but I also think that's not exactly what she meant.

The truth, of course, is that I'm having a lot *more* fun these days than I ever did back when people may have been more likely to associate me with the word. Mostly because I'm a generally happier person than I ever have been before, and also because I honestly think that StoryTime Hour at the children's library followed by a playdate that includes cheese puffs for the short people and wine for the tall ones makes for kind of the best day ever.

The other night I was paging through *US Weekly* and came across a photo of Demi Moore and Lenny Kravitz at a club . . . and you know what stood out to me the most? That the photo was taken at 1:30 a.m. And my jaw basically unhinged itself in awe at the disconnect between their lives and mine, despite the fact that they're both parents, and both quite a bit older than I am.

That I got all pearls-clutch-y "oh, my . . . but that's so *late!*" about this photo is nuts, when I consider what I was up to just a few years ago. Closing down bars, dancing on tables, seeing sunrises . . . none of these things were unusual on a Tuesday. I've talked about my twenties being everything from lonely to troubled—and they were those things, yes, yes—but they were also *wild*. If you catch me in just the right, overshare-y mood, I've got some pretty crazy stories to tell.

And! I don't think there's anything wrong with being out late, with partying (responsibly; let's stick to moderate amounts of legal substances and stay far away from wheels), or with Demi Moore flirting with Lenny Kravitz (hey, I would, and Kendrick would understand why, because the man is *cute*). I just don't want to do it. Like . . . ever. The things I enjoy doing these days—getting up early to eat pancakes at a diner with my family, watching episode after episode of *American Horror Story* until the ungodly hour of 11:00 p.m., grabbing dinner with some girlfriends, fixing up our house—are fulfilling and exciting to me now in the way that finding the best after-party used to be.

When I think back on what I was doing, I realize that I was trying to fill a hole. A hole that's filled now. I'm not saying that's what everyone is doing when they're going out and getting a little rowdy—not at all; I think in many ways it's an important part of the growing-up, boundary-pushing process—but that is definitely what I was up to. My life felt purposeless, out-of-control, solitary . . . and when I was sitting in a bar with people I had just met but who suddenly felt like my best! friends! ever! . . . well, I felt better in some ways. And worse, of course, in others.

But I still worry, sometimes. Because that girl who I used to be, just so you know, is the same girl who my husband met on MySpace all those years ago. And lately . . . I've changed. A lot. And sometmes I wonder whether that's okay.

I've figured out, I think, where a lot of this worry comes from: For a couple of years in my mid-twenties I dated a guy who was very into going out, and did go out pretty much every single night. A year or so into our relationship, I started to realize that I didn't *want* to go out all the time; that a night in with a movie and takeout—just the two of us, relaxing at home and maybe even, I don't know, talking (!)—was starting to sound not just like a nice change, but completely wonderful. A necessary evolution, in fact, if our relationship was ever going to be more than what it was. But when I suggested that we start staying in once in awhile, what he said to me was this: "If you get boring, that's going to be a real problem." In other words: You better act like my crazy twenty-five-year-old girlfriend in the very specific ways that I want you to for the rest of your life, or I am outta here.

He was not a very good boyfriend. This is a pretty good example of why we broke up.

I'm more than aware that "going out" doesn't equate with being "fun" or "exciting," and that my ex had somewhat flawed priorities, but that conversation still pops up in my head once in a while. And I still worry, you know: Is it okay with my husband that he met and fell in love with one person . . . and now, seven years later, wakes up to someone else entirely? I'm sure that some part of him misses the girl who used to be more than happy to play darts until four in the morning, but I also feel relatively certain that the things he got when that girl started shape-shifting back into who she truly was are things that he likes even better.

I think what it comes down to is this: Life changes, and people change right along with it. And that's a good thing. But there are some things that don't change, that *can't*, and those are the things that the ones who care about you love the very most. It wasn't the crazy party girl that Kendrick fell in love with; it was the crazy party girl that he *liked*. The person he fell in love with was someone very different, someone who was just trying a "party girl" persona on for size for a little while.

I didn't fall in love with a guy in a rock band who looked cool onstage. Sure, I liked going to see my husband's band play on tour, liked it when he winked at me from the stage; all that was so much fun . . . but I fell in love with a guy who once filled 365 note-cards with things he thought were great about me and then sealed them in envelopes so that I could open one every single day for an entire year. I also didn't fall in love with him because of grand gestures like that; I fell in love with him because he has a heart that makes such gestures possible.

You know who I feel the most like these days? The person I was in elementary school: the kid who liked writing and reading, and who mostly just wanted to hang out with her family.

Parties are fun and exciting and all that . . . but the best party, right now, is right here in our living room: It involves footie PJs, apple pie, and figuring out how, exactly, to say the word *hippopotamus*. That's what I call a wild night.

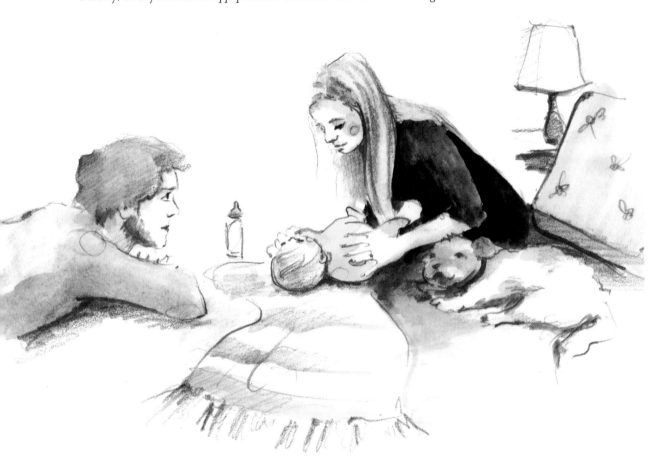

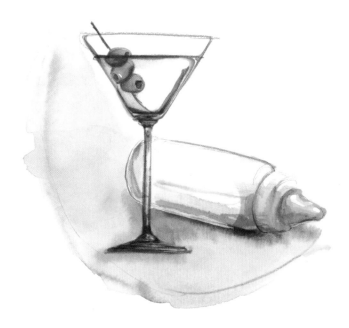

Getting Out

(Your Baby Is Amazing and Super-Cute, But Not Everyone in the World Is Going to Agree with You on That One)

That Couple That Ruins It for Everyone

About a month after we became parents, my husband and I decided to go on our first Date Night. We left our son with my mother, I got dressed up in a very strange outfit involving a see-through white fringe top, silver sparkle shorts, and suede knee-high boots (the idea of going out in public post–7:00 p.m. and mingling with actual adults apparently got me so overexcited that I completely forgot how to get dressed), and we walked two whole blocks away to a romantic brick-walled gastropub that served things like expensive burgers and cocktails with oversized ice cubes in them. We settled down at our table, held hands, and laughed a little at how strange it felt to be out in the "normal" world again, and started doing what it turns out most parents do when presented with a night out on the town away from their children: talking about our child.

Then we noticed the couple at the next table. They were that very particular kind of cool that immediately identified them as the kind of people who probably spend Saturday mornings at art galleries before returning home to play their banjos while sitting on the steps of their Brooklyn townhouse. The guy was wearing a fedora and had bunches of tattoos, the girl was wearing big jewelry and a patterned skirt, and they were sitting at a long wooden table surrounded by a bunch of equally stylish friends. They were also accompanied by a very small baby—maybe three months old—who was planted on her dad's lap, occasionally drawing attention because of something adorable she'd done but mostly flying under the radar. At one point the dad got up and tossed the baby in the air and she giggled, and Kendrick and I literally *oohed* and *aahed*. Literally. I think I said "Ooh!" and Kendrick said "Aah."

It was that cute.

It was also a wildly unfortunate scene for a new set of parents to come across.

"Look at them!" we said to each other, eyes all glowy and naïve. "Let's be *just like them*. Let's take the baby out to dinner with us all the time, wherever we want to go, and he'll get used to being out in public so fast that he'll be super-calm and easygoing no matter what! It'll be amazing."

I continue to think that what happened on that Date Night was that we stumbled upon one of those rare moments of total calm and ease that does occasionally happen even to the very greenest of parents. The problem when something like a child smiling happily through a multi-course meal occurs in public, though, is that it makes all the other parents who bear witness either terribly jealous or dangerously reckless. They start thinking that they, too, should take their infant out to the awesome new restaurant down the block. "Sure," they say to themselves, "it doesn't seem like a place that's particularly kid-friendly, but hey: we'll make it work!"

They get cocky.

I had one of those moments myself the other night, when I took my son out to a sushi dinner. It was just the two of us, sitting there having a nice little chat ("That?" "Car." "That?" "It's a car." "That?" "Still a car.") and eating tempura. Doesn't that sound lovely and refined?

It *was* lovely and refined. I'm serious: My son was the absolute picture of Sweet Adorable Child from start to finish. He enthusiastically ate things that he'd never tried before, smiled and cried out "See you!" at the waitress, diligently applied himself to the challenge of figuring out how a pair of kids' chopsticks work (and succeeding in using them to transmit a piece of broccoli—broccoli!—from plate to mouth), placed his napkin gently on the table alongside his dish, and was so generally pleasant and well-behaved that I was complimented on my stellar parenting by not one, but *two* people.

Two people called me a good parent. Unprovoked!

My experience with parenting comments delivered by total strangers, incidentally, is more along the lines of "You are creating irreparable damage to your child by doing X," so to say this whole event left me a little taken aback is an understatement.

But like I said: The problem when moments like this happen is that they can make you cocky, and cocky is bad. You start thinking, "Oh man, I totally got this." You do things like leave the house without an extra diaper, because it was cool that one time. (Do not ever, *ever* leave the house without an extra diaper. I do this frequently because I'm a space cadet and I never learn . . . but I am also the one flailing around in the playground using my sleeve as a tissue, if you recall, so do as I say, et cetera.)

Back to that tattooed, fedora-ed couple and how they inspired us to take our son out to dinner. A few days later, we packed up the diaper bag and the three of us headed out to a nearby Mexican place that we figured would be more or less empty at the early (in New York City) hour of 5:00 p.m. Our son was quiet and wide-eyed and happy for the entire stroller ride, and we took our time getting there, holding hands and snuggling a little while we walked and thinking, Wow, this parenting thing is so *easy*.

Our son started screaming his tiny head off the moment we stepped foot into the restaurant. The only way to put the circus on pause was to basically do high-kicks around the room with our child in tow. Oh, and forget about sitting down and/or consuming food. Don't you dare take that bite, Dad: I will see you, and I will be *furious*.

Eventually, the very nice young lady who had taken our order came over and asked us if we would like her to hold our son for a while so that we could actually eat. We declined, deciding that waitress intervention was probably a good indicator that we should leave an enormous tip and get out of there immediately.

Anyway, best laid plans and so on.

Later on there were dinners that went better, and even many, many dinners that went *great*—that were far more fun, in fact, than any dinner we'd had in our pre-parent lives—but still, what we learned is this: While kids don't put a halt to your ability to do the things that you want to do . . . they do require you to make a few small compromises. Be a little more unflappable. Abandon all vestiges of self-consciousness.

Take a chill pill.

An Angry Infant for You, a Martini for Me

My husband is so nice. I mean that. He is a really, truly, honestly *nice man*, and a much, much nicer person than I could ever hope to be. In the early months after our son was born, as an example, he responded to the fact that I was completely overwhelmed and so exhausted that I could barely even speak by the time 6:00 p.m. rolled around by suggesting that we "go grab a drink."

Now, you can't just "go grab a drink" with a baby. Or at least not with an awake baby. Not with *our* awake baby, in any case.

So what my husband meant by "let's go grab a drink" was this: He would deposit me at a restaurant on Second Avenue, put our son into the stroller, and walk him and walk him and walk him until he finally fell asleep, at which point he would join me, take the last sip of my martini, and then accompany me to the ice cream shop, where he'd buy me a cone.

Like I said: a nice, nice man.

The point of this story, though, is not just that I don't deserve my husband (although I don't): It's also that sometimes what you want to do—go relax together at a restaurant, have a conversation that lasts for more than five minutes, and eat or drink something while seated—might simply not be possible for the time being. A lot of it, of course, depends on circumstances. Every child is different, and every family handles those differences in their own way.

What's important is that you find workarounds—whether that's one of you taking your baby for a walk around the block while the other takes a break for a moment, or ordering in Chinese and having a coffee-table picnic in front of a good movie after the baby falls asleep, or trying out a new restaurant during brunch rather than dinner—that make you feel like you're still getting to do the things that you love to do, and that make you feel relaxed and happy and like yourself. You still get to do what you want . . . you just have to be a little less specific about what that means. You have to get a little more creative.

As an example, if going out to eat is something that's important to you—if it's a big part of your life, and an activity that you don't want to give up even when your child is very young—you can make it work. You just have to make it work for *everyone* to the greatest extent possible . . .

And remember that "everyone" isn't just the three of you; it's the rest of the world out there. They count, too.

Restaurants and Babies

The topic of when and how (and whether) you should bring small children out to restaurants is apparently a controversial one. I get why, because both sides of the argument make sense: On the one hand, there should indeed be places where a person can consume a meal without the accompanying strains of *Yo Gabba Gabba!* on an iPad somewhere in the background. There are places where napkins should stay on laps, Cheerios should not accidentally end up on floors, and food should be eaten with utensils.

In short: There are restaurants that should be exclusively for adults. This is true.

On the other side of the Restaurants and Babies argument are those who believe that children are actually small people as opposed to mildly self-aware amoebas, and should thus be permitted to go places—like restaurants—where people go. They feel that they are entitled to bring their family members out into the world if they so choose, and also feel that it's good for children to be exposed to a wide range of situations (including those in which they are expected to comport themselves in a relatively controlled manner).

Restaurants can be excellent—and fun—experiences for children. This is true also.

What it really comes down to, though, is whether *you* want to go. If you honestly would prefer to discover the new Thai place in town in the exclusive company of adults, that's perfectly fine . . . but if it's important for you to find ways to bring the kids out with you, that's doable as well; you just need to keep a few things in mind.

Let's talk how to get out and go.

How-To: TAKE A BABY TO A RESTAURANT

CHOOSE WISELY. When it comes to kids and restaurants, it's all about location and timing. Err on the side of "casual" and "early": You certainly don't need to restrict yourself to Chuck E. Cheese's and McDonald's . . . but if you want to try out that cool new Argentinian place down the block, try going right when it opens and is relatively empty. And remember: There are some places—places with, say, tasting menus that cost upward of $100 per plate—where kids just don't mix. That's what Date Nights are for.

WHAT TO LOOK FOR WHEN CHOOSING A RESTAURANT

- AMBIENT NOISE. Silence is not a friend of the couple who travels with children. Some music over the loudspeakers disguises mini-tantrums (and high-decibel shrieks of joy) nicely.

- FUN STUFF TO LOOK AT. We love hibachi restaurants because the chefs put on a performance that keeps our son entertained while we chat. Anywhere with live music, cool decorations, or paper tablecloths that come complete with cups of crayons is a good bet.

- FAST SERVICE. Don't be afraid to let your server know that you'd appreciate your order being taken as quickly as possible . . . or bring along some snacks to portion out while you wait for your food to arrive.

- FRIENDLY WAITSTAFF. Some of my favorite places to go out are my favorites because the servers are just so *great* and so clearly enjoy having kids around. Places (and people) like this are treasures, and should be rewarded appropriately, with repeat patronage and large tips.

BRING REINFORCEMENTS. I don't believe that children should be coddled within an inch of their lives and kept entertained 100 percent of the time lest they grow frustrated. Frustration is a normal part of the human experience, and something that everyone must learn to cope with. In restaurants, I become the biggest hypocrite on this point that you have ever seen: I will give my child whatever he needs—whether that's a toy, a book, constant food delivery, or a full-on song-and-dance Mama Spectacular—in order to avoid even the slightest whisper of irritation. Why? Because while I want my family to have a good time, I also want to make sure that our little adventure doesn't intrude on the enjoyment of my fellow diners.

TREAT YOUR SERVER LIKE A PERSON. Just because you have a child with you does not give you the right to act like a bossypants. Dining out with a baby can be stressful, but that was your decision; you're certainly entitled to request, say, a speedy delivery of a bread basket or a straw to go with your daughter's glass of juice, but remember: One of the reasons that you're taking your child out in the first place is to expose him to things in the world you want him to be exposed to . . . like manners. Set a good example.

KEEP IT CLEAN. Part of the fun of eating out is not having to do the heavy lifting (cooking, washing dishes, et cetera), and certainly everyone understands that kids can get a little messy. But back to using the experience as a positive example for your child: No one is expecting you to Fantastik the floor, but taking a moment before you leave to quickly pick up any major offenders lets the employees know that you appreciate their work and respect their space.

KNOW WHEN TO MAKE AN EXIT. Sometimes babies cry. And yell. And throw stuff. These things happen, and if they happen in a restaurant there's no need to freak out. Just be as courteous of others as possible, and do what you can to put an end to the disturbance. That said, there are times when you need to cut your losses and leave. Any instance involving, say, projectile vomit, ear-piercing shrieks that will not stop, or one of those terrible floor-collapse tantrum things are all good indicators that it is time to pay and go. Now. (You'll get dessert next time.)

- **BRING OUT THE YUMMIES.** I don't know what it is about cheese sticks, but they apparently taste like chocolate-covered heaven on toast. The second one comes out, it's all hands on cheese, and that is a good thing.

- **STAGE A SURPRISE.** I keep small, inexpensive toy cars that my son has never seen before in my purse, and pull them out when I feel a meltdown coming.

In short: Every child has a food or toy Achilles' heel. Have that heel in your purse.

ICE THAT PASTA

As it turns out, the ability to delay gratification is a learned skill. Perhaps it shows up at some point in Year Two; I don't know, we're not there yet. All I know is that when a waiter plonks down a bowl of macaroni and cheese in front of my son, it is going directly in his mouth regardless of temperature. And if it's too hot, we have tears . . . but not tears quite as loud as those that will be unleashed should the too-hot food be placed out of reach so that it may cool.

See food = Put food in mouth. That's just how this equation works.

I always request that our server allow my son's dish to cool in the kitchen for a minute before bringing it out, but if that doesn't happen there's nothing a quick stir with a few ice cubes can't fix. Sure, it'll water down the end product a little, but that's a small price to pay for a happily unburned (and occupied) little tongue.

Hotels and Babies

The summer that my son was a year and a half old, I decided that it was time to get rid of the pacifier that he was still using for naps and at bedtime. The prospect of going back to the era of waking up multiple times a night with a restless baby really stressed me out, though, so what did I do?

I made sure that I took my son's pacifier away the day before we left on a family trip in which we were all staying together in a single (small) hotel room, of course! Because we all know that the best thing to do when you are altering a major part of a child's routine is to make sure that all the other parts—like the part where he sleeps at home, in his bedroom, alone—are thrown into upheaval as well.

Clearly.

The first night in that hotel room was not good. At eight p.m., Kendrick and I put our son in his Pack n Play and turned off the lights, and then got under the covers and essentially hid from him, trying to read our Kindles without showing any sign of life. It was exactly as relaxing and fun as it sounds, and worked not at all. The pacifier wasn't the problem; the problem was that Mom and Dad were right there, doing exciting things like being awake. Our son stood straight up in his crib staring at us for two full hours, after which we finally decided to give up and shut the party down.

The next night, though? Pretty good.

And the night after that was actually . . . yes, relaxing. All we needed, as it turned out, was to make a few small tweaks to any ideas about "vacation" that we had held in our previous, non-parent lives, and all was well.

How-To: HIT UP A HOTEL WITH A BABY

MAKE IT HOMEY. Most hotels will provide a Pack n Play (or similar), but it's a good idea to bring along your own sheets and a blanket, as well as a much-loved stuffed animal, to try to approximate the feeling of your child's sleeping space at home as closely as possible.

MINIMIZE DISTRACTIONS. Set up the crib in a dark, quiet corner, and position a smartphone or tablet loaded with a white noise app nearby to cut out ambient noise.

STOCK UP ON SNACKS. Even if you're planning to eat all your meals in restaurants, make sure the in-room refrigerator is decently well-stocked: Handing over a little juice and yogurt first thing in the morning will give you the leeway you need to get ready to head out for the day.

KEEP IT CONSISTENT. Try to stick to the same naptime schedule you use at home. That may mean trucking back to your hotel at midday and hanging out while your child rests, and that may not be ideal . . . but I'm not sure you've seen "not ideal" until you've seen an unnapped toddler who is being asked to sit calmly in his stroller through half an hour of Mom checking out that atmospherically cluttered antique store in which *nothing must be touched* (speaking from experience). Look for ways to make those breaks in the day fun: One partner can go for a run or check out the town while the other stays in the room, and then you can switch off the next day.

NIGHT NIGHT! If you're all staying in the same room, your bedtime is basically the same as your kids' (unless they're able to sleep with things going on around them; mine isn't). Once they've fallen asleep you can read, play a quiet board game with the lights low, or—my personal favorite option—sneak a bottle of wine and some junk food into the room and have a picnic on the bedspread.

STAY TUNED. Bring along a baby monitor. If you don't feel like sitting in the bedroom after lights-out, the monitor will give you the freedom to hang out on the porch (or in the bathtub).

RELAX AND ENJOY. Traveling with kids is stressful, but it's also kind of the best. Find your Zen place, and don't forget those cheese sticks.

Movies and Babies

All right, not going to lie: Taking a child under the age of two to a full-length movie in a for-real movie theater is some serious business.

Sure, it might be easier to just wait a couple of years, until they're old enough to understand the concept of "movie = Gummi Bears and joy" . . . but you know what I think? Provided you follow some basic Laws of Common Sense and Respect for Your Fellow Moviegoer (see below), this is a to-each-his-own situation. We really love the movies, and our son seems to really love them as well, so off to the theater we go.

How-To: SEE A MOVIE WITH A TODDLER

KNOW YOUR CHILD. Some kids can sit (relatively) still. Some cannot. If yours is the latter, maybe hold off for a little while; there's no use making all of you miserable during an activity that's supposed to be fun.

PICK THE RIGHT TIME. Not naptime.

GET PREPPED. For example, if you know that a kids' movie about trains is coming out, spend some time during the week prior getting your child excited about the subject matter. Watch mini-movies about trains on YouTube, look at pictures of them in books, and generally try to wind up to the grand finale (which would be the movie).

THE EMPTIER THE THEATER, THE BETTER. Ideally, you want to pick a morning matinee of a movie that's been out for a while (and there's no rule that says that popcorn and Raisinets cannot be consumed at 10:30 a.m.).

BE FASHIONABLY LATE. You know what previews are? Fifteen fewer minutes that your child will be able to watch the feature. Plan to show up to the theater at the time that the movie is scheduled to begin; by the time you've gotten your tickets and concessions the previews will have finished.

SELECT YOUR SEAT. Find an empty side row, and sit at the outside edge (right next to the aisle) with your child between you and the wall: It creates a contained space for him to move around in the event he gets fidgety.

SNACKS, SNACKS, SNACKS. Bring more snacks than you can possibly imagine going into the body of one small human over the course of an hour and a half, and then bring more. Bring options. Bring drinks. And do not bring them out all at once. Wait as long as you can before even introducing the idea of food and/or beverages, and then distribute them as slowly as possible.

HAVE SOME (SILENT) TOYS. I keep a handful of small toys in my purse all the time, and during the expository lull in a movie's second act I hand them over so that our son can play with them for a few minutes while he waits for the action to pick back up.

KNOW WHEN TO MAKE AN EXIT. Screaming = time to go. Now. (You'll catch the rest on Netflix.)

Babies on a Plane

If both parents are not present at the time that a child is issued a United States passport, the absent parent must provide a notarized Statement of Consent prior to the issuance of said travel document.

I totally knew that, which is a minor miracle in and of itself. I was uncharacteristically responsible and read it on the Internet before heading over to the post office, so when I handed in my son's passport application I also had that (notarized!) Statement of Consent from my husband in hand.

I did not, however, know that were I to then fly to Canada with my son and without my husband, I would need to bring along a *second* letter of permission in order to gain entry to the country. It's a rule that makes sense—yes, let's please keep parents from traveling internationally with their children without letting the child's other parent know—but still: It's not a fun fact to learn while standing in a very small, very bright, very windowless room with a five-month-old baby at two o'clock in the morning.

I was headed to Moncton, a smallish city located near Canada's Eastern seaboard, to visit my aunts and cousins for a few days. It was the first time I was taking a flight with my son—something I was *extremely* nervous about to begin with—and the already stressful undertaking concluded rather spectacularly, with a Canadian Border Patrol officer making the following phone call to my husband:

"Hello, sir. This is Officer X of the Canadian Border Patrol. Do you know where your wife and child are?"

. . . Pause while my husband presumably lost ten years of his life to a heart attack.

"Are you aware that they boarded a flight to Canada this evening?"

Another pause. Ten more years.

It took the officer a good five minutes to reach the point in the conversation where he alerted my husband to the fact that his wife and child were both alive and not presently located in a jail, hospital, asylum, fire station, interrogation booth, and/or torture chamber. I'm sure this is protocol, and the officer was very kind and professional through the entire encounter, but I'm also sure that this was not a pleasant experience for my husband (and also entirely my fault).

In short: Flying with children is guaranteed to be something of a drama, so let's just accept that fact and go from there.

The next time I flew with my son was when my husband and I decided to take a vacation to the Dominican Republic when he was just over a year and a half old. On the morning that we left, everything went so smoothly that I could hardly believe it. I remembered to bring our passports *and* immunization records, no wayward letters of permission were required, and our son passed the car ride to the airport happily rotating through the series of travel-appropriate snacks that we'd toted along in little see-through containers.

Now, can we all agree that—whether you have a child or not—going through airport security is straight-up *terrible*? No matter how prepared you are—belt off, jewelry removed, laptop out of bag—it's like a madcap panic-dash of misery. Add a toddler who is just starting to realize that he is in a completely unfamiliar, fluorescent place and that he is actually supposed to be mid-nap *right now*—and boom: it's a quick elevator ride down to that seventh circle.

So yes, airport security is always terrible . . . but this time it was extra terrible, because I had an increasingly cranky toddler in my arms, and when I went to retrieve my bag from the conveyer belt and slip on my sandals two things happened simultaneously:

1. The strap holding my shoe on my foot snapped.
2. The strap holding my handbag on my shoulder fell off.

These things happened at the *same exact moment*. I know, you think I'm lying. I'm totally not.

My husband was still mid-madcap security panic-dash himself, so I sort of hop-limped over to a bench to begin the process of figuring out how to put myself back together in a way that would enable me to move, because with a baby, a flappy shoe, and a bag that had transformed into an extremely heavy bowling ball . . . I couldn't. I sat there on the bench with my now-apoplectic son on my lap, staring at the panorama of Things That I Could Not Fix strewn about me, and do you know what happened?

A man came walking over, patted me on the shoulder, and said, "I have two daughters. Traveling with kids is really difficult, and I just want you to know that I think you're doing a good job."

It was the nicest thing I could possibly have heard at that moment (other than, perhaps, "Hello, here is a new pair of shoes and a bag with a strap").

That's the first thing to remember when traveling with a child: It's an undertaking that *everyone* dreads, and everyone (everyone who is a parent, at least) is deeply sympathetic to that fact. They're rooting for you. They're rooting for your kid. They want to see you make it through with your sanity intact . . . and if they can help you, they probably will.

There are, however, a few things that you can do to make the whole process easier on all involved.

How-To: MAKE IT THROUGH A FLIGHT WITH A BABY

DON'T FREAK OUT. Try to find your own personal Zen Place: If you're anxious and upset, the baby will pick up on it and get worked up in turn.

KNOW YOU'RE NOT THE FIRST. The flight attendants have experienced crying babies on planes before, and (a) feel bad for you, and (b) will do what they can to assist. Ask them for suggestions. Ask them if you can hang out in the aisle and bounce the baby for a while. Ask them for a hug; they'll probably give you one.

MAKE A (VISIBLE) EFFORT. We all know that there are times when children will not stop crying whatever you do, but now is not the time to shrug and go back to your book while your kid slams his feet into the seat in front of him. Even if you suspect your efforts will be in vain, looking like you're at least trying to find a solution does wonders.

SNACKS AND SNACKS AND MORE SNACKS. Have so many snacks. Then have more.

BRING A CARRIER. You can use a baby carrier to get through security— they probably won't make you take it off—and then call it into action for some midflight rocking, if need be.

DIVIDE AND CONQUER. Let your traveling partner board first to stow your carry-ons, and then wait to board with the baby until the last possible second. The more time you can spend getting energy out preflight, the better.

OFFER BOTTLE SERVICE. Provide a bottle during takeoff and landing to help your baby's ears clear.

BREAK OUT THE SURPRISES. Pack a couple of inexpensive, brand-new toys, and pull them out to head off any especially fussy moments.

STICK TO A SCHEDULE. Of course you'll have to be improvisational, but as much as you can, try to stick to your normal routine: Put your child into his PJs at the regular time; bring the stuffed animal he's used to sleeping with on the plane; try to approximate his pre-bedtime routine as much as possible.

OWN (OR BORROW) AN IPAD. That's all.

Above all: Don't stress if things don't go perfectly. An in-transit baby may not be a happy baby, but it's just a few hours. You'll make it through.

Entertaining at Home

I'll be honest: Historically, I've tended to be a little show-offy when people come over. I like to use fancy china, put out adorable little appetizer things, and generally find ways to make my guests *ooh* and *aah* so that I can bask in the glow of my impressive homemaker-ness.

I am extremely unimpressive these days.

Or, rather: I may still *appear* (marginally) impressive to the casually observant guest, but now I'm all deceptive and underhanded about it. I cheat.

Here's the thing: The amount of time that I have in my life to sit down with a glass of wine and communicate with other human adults has dwindled considerably since the arrival in my home of a person who spent the first year of his life requiring my constant attention and care for mere survival. And that's fine; I would rather spend time with him than with anyone else on the planet. When I *do* get the chance to relax with friends for a bit, though, the last thing I want to be doing is running around all chicken-with-my-head-cut-off, whipping up from-scratch brownies and cutting carrots into pretty garnish shapes or whatever it is that I used to do.

These days, I want to make life a little easier on myself.

EASY ENTERTAINING SHORTCUTS

When you have guests over, you can make everything from scratch and plate all the courses just-so and make yourself crazy . . . or you can cut corners in a few simple ways that streamline the whole process *enormously*.

HORS D'OEUVRES. Do not make them. Buy them. If they're removed from the plastic containers that they came in and set on pretty dishes, chances are no one will ever know the difference (or care).

CHEESE. Cheese is a home entertainer's little miracle. All you have to do is pick up a few interesting varieties and some crackers, stick them on a chalkboard serving plate and write the names of the cheeses next to them, and there you go: You have a conversation piece that looks like it just flew right off of a Pinterest board.

DIPS. Pour store-bought dips into serving bowls, and then top them with pretty, unexpected garnishes (try a little arugula, chopped red pepper, or a few capers sprinkled over a dish of hummus).

DRINKS. Forget the full bar. All you really need is some wine, beer, and a couple of nonalcoholic options.

SWEETS. Instantly make a boxed cake look like a dessert you spent hours slaving over by cutting it into tiers and filling the center with (store-bought) whipped cream and fresh berries. Or put out Yodels, because Yodels are magical.

When it comes to serving, here's what I want you to do: Sit. Down. Set out the food and drinks on buffet tables along with stacks of dishes and cups filled with cutlery, and let your guests serve themselves. Then, when everyone's done eating and that nice guest or two offers to help clear the table or do a few dishes? Graciously say "thank you" . . . and then let them help. Help is good.

IF LOTS OF KIDS ARE ON THE GUEST LIST...

One more thing to remember when entertaining at home, especially if you're having a multiple-child-inclusive party: Accidents are going to happen. Some ways to keep the damage to a minimum:

- If you're planning to have kids of a variety of ages hanging around, remember to look for potential problems at every height level—actually get down on your hands and knees and check out your home from the perspective of a baby, a toddler, and a child to see what hazards you may have overlooked.

- Consider using pretty paper or plastic plates, cups, and cutlery instead of the good stuff; honestly, you can find versions that are absolutely gorgeous, and easy cleanup = happy hostess.

- If you insist on using real wine glasses, at least go for stemless ones that are less likely to tip over.

- This is not the time or the place to break out Grandma's china; a good rule of thumb is to not put out anything at all that would make you cry were it to break.

- Abandon all TV-related morality systems. If you have a bunch of verging-on-bored little people milling about but the grown-ups want to keep hanging out for a while longer, nothing saves the day like Pixar. Nothing.

Damn It, It's Raining Again
(At-Home Activities)

When I was in fourth grade, I had a pet bird named Tango and a Maine Coon cat named Duncan. Tango was a little yellow cockatiel who liked to hang out on top of his cage, whipping Duncan into a frenzy by virtue of his very out-of-reach existence and occasionally taking little trips across the room to perch on my shoulder.

One day I was sitting on the floor playing Tetris when I heard an enormous crash coming from the general direction of Tango's cage. I ran over, only to discover that Duncan—who was not a small cat, by the way—had somehow catapulted himself three feet up into the air and straight through the (very, very tiny) door of the birdcage. After a speedy, frantic search we found Tango sitting under the couch, appropriately freaked out but essentially unharmed. Duncan wasn't so lucky: As excited as he must have been to discover that he was capable of launching himself into the birdcage, he was slightly less excited to discover that he was going to have a hell of a time getting himself back out.

A cat trapped in a birdcage is not a happy cat.

That's sort of what rainy days at home with a toddler are like. The best way to handle them: get busy, and get busy *quickly*.

Three of my favorite (free!) at-home activity ideas:

TEXTURE TABLE

Just look around the house for a bunch of items with varying textures (try leaves, pinecones, grass, marshmallows, plastic spoons, raisins, silky scarves, and cotton balls, keeping in mind not to incorporate things that are too small if your toddler is still in the everything-goes-in-my-mouth stage, and to monitor closely regardless) and spread them out on the floor or on a large, unbreakable plate. A small plastic cup is a nice addition, as it can be used both as a receptacle and as a pouring device.

> Remember that playing with grains and other very small objects of which there are thousands can get a little messy, so don't set up shop in an area where spillage will make you nuts.

OBSTACLE COURSE

Create an at-home play gym using dining room chairs, pillows, stuffed animals, end tables, and anything else your toddler can climb under, around, over, or through. While for-real playgrounds are nice and all . . . there's something even more fun about climbing over the pillows from your living room couch.

BASKET OF JOY

Pile a ton of age-appropriate household items (scarves, hats, mixing spoons, Tupperware, et cetera) into a laundry basket, and let your kid go to town.

Mama Friendships and Making the Time

When we first moved out of the city, I knew exactly no one in our new town except for the woman who had sold us our house. My first few weeks were filled with unpacking, organizing, cleaning, and aimlessly wandering the streets in search of places where one might take an eleven-month-old to have a really killer time.

Everywhere I looked I saw women strollering around with kids about my son's age, but the mere sight of these groups of moms—all of whom were obviously best friends with each other already—immediately transported me back to second grade. Suddenly, there I was: sitting on a beach somewhere with my mom pushing me toward the girl about my age who was playing in the sand nearby and telling me to just *go say hi already*.

Never in my life—either prior to having a baby or since—have I been possessed of the desire to go up to a total stranger and say hi.

But when I moved, I had to get over this little hang-up nice and quick if I didn't want to spend the rest of my life in the Mommy and Me equivalent of solitary confinement.

Buddies and Babies

One of the best side effects of writing a blog is that it has made me work much, much harder to figure out the reality behind situations that initially feel unmanageable—mostly because I spend a lot of time circling around problems in my head before ever sitting down to write.

I know exactly what's going on with this thing that's on my mind right now. But knowing what's going on and being able to understand it are two different matters.

I love watching my son and my husband playing. I love how much they love each other; I love what an incredible father Kendrick is; I love how completely obsessed our son is with every single thing that Kendrick says and does. But in the past couple of weeks something new has happened, and it's that my son no longer wants very much to do with me when his dad is around. He wants daddy to pick him up, wants daddy to play with him. He cries when Kendrick takes so much as a step into the other room, and having me hold him instead doesn't seem to be a comfort. When Kendrick isn't around it's totally business as usual—snuggling, lots of "lah doo Mama" (that's "love you Mommy" in toddler-speak), laughing and playing and wonderful . . . but when Kendrick comes home at the end of the day, my son jumps straight out of my arms and into my husband's.

I understand this completely. I know what I would say to a reader if she wrote this to me in an email.

"Children go through phases, and it's completely normal for them to want to be with one parent more than another for a period of time. It doesn't mean that they love you any less, and it doesn't have grand, far-reaching implications. It makes sense that it hurts, but you need to focus on the reality, and the reality is that you're dealing with a toddler who loves you unconditionally and whose actions are not necessarily reflective of his feelings or intentions."

I know all of this, and it still crushes me when my baby is crying and my arms aren't enough to make him stop.

And I can't talk to Kendrick about it, because his response—understandably—is to tell me that our son loves me, and of course I know that. And hearing someone try to "convince" me of it makes me feel simultaneously silly and sad and disappointed in myself for even needing to talk about this at all.

Yesterday morning, I sat down to email my friend Morgan (who used to live just down the street from me in New York City and now lives across the country with her husband and two children) and started to update her about work and life and blah blah blah . . . and then I stopped, deleted it all, and wrote this:

Hi! My son loves Kendrick more than he loves me.

How are you?

I knew that she would know that I was simultaneously kidding and a little bummed out, and what she wrote back was not how to "fix things" or that "everything is fine," but rather—in essence—"oh my god me *too*." Which was exactly what I needed to hear.

These past few weeks, I've been lonely. A little loneliness comes with the self-employed territory, and is just one small negative in a whole field of positives, but it's still not the best feeling in the world. I realized this a couple of weeks ago, when I pulled off the road into a farmstand and bought myself a bouquet just because it was pretty, and almost cried when I realized that I was actually buying it because I felt very alone and thought that flowers might make feeling alone feel better.

Lately, for whatever reason, it's just felt easier to stay in, to get through the workday and then play with my son and watch TV and then fall asleep and get up and do it all over again, rarely exchanging more than a handful of non-emailed sentences with someone over the age of two. But I think that it's important—essential, even—that I try to push back against this, because I can tell that something about this mini self-imposed isolation is what's making it hard for me to handle my son reaching away from me—a thing that he will (and should) do countless times as he grows and becomes more and more independent.

I've heard all the "it's hard to make friends when you're a parent" talk, but it's more than that: Yes, it's super hard to make friends as a parent . . . but it's also easy to forget that you need friends at all. You prioritize family (of course), and work (of course), and put off that drink or that dinner until next week, next month, when you have a little more time (which ends up being never). I need to make the time.

Making friends as a grown-up is a tough business (I personally spend approximately 90 percent of my first conversation with a new person trying to figure out exactly how much of my personality I can reveal while not freaking them out), and making friends as a new mom can be even tougher. Sure, it's easier in some ways—you have built-in reasons called "children" to get together, and can use playdate time to figure out whether you have anything in common other than the fact that you have both recently procreated—but adding things like kids who may or may not whack each other in the face and widely variable attitudes toward child-rearing can also throw a major curveball of apprehension into each and every encounter. The point of friendship is theoretically to enjoy each other's company and help each other get through the hard stuff, and being a parent is nothing if not hard . . . but still: Navigating those early conversations with another parent can feel like tip-toeing through a minefield of possible ways to offend.

So what do you talk about with a New Mom Friend? You talk about your children, of course (because really, at this point having children is the one thing you know you have in common). You also want to seem "cool" and not talk constantly about your children . . . but then worry that if you don't talk constantly about your children you will appear to be a terrible mother. Then you say something vaguely opinionated (aka "interesting") and worry that you've just made a statement that will stand in total opposition to the value system of the other mom present and cause a grievous and potential-friendship-ending offense . . . but of course you also want to show that you're not offended by anything *she* might say, so you get all self-deprecating and weird and forget it: Now you've alienated her completely, having cycled through about twenty-six different personalities in the time it takes to drink a single cup of coffee.

It's like dating, except there's a baby present and a decent chance that you're too tired to form full sentences.

Starting from scratch in a brand-new town with a brand-new child, a brand-new home, and a brand-new life, I was a big old ball of anxiety, and could barely gather the courage to say hi to the mom in line next to me at the grocery store—forget about trying to set up a playdate. But then, as time went on, all those nerves started to wear on me . . . and then started to wear right out, as I realized that not only was the vast majority of the judgment all in my head (just as it had been on that beach in second grade) . . . the part of it that was real? *Didn't matter.*

When it comes to making for-real new friends as an adult and as a parent, the first thing to remember is this: Everyone is just as worried about how they measure up as you are. In fact, it's more than likely that all the other moms you meet are so worried that you'll deem their parenting skills appalling because they're handing over Chef Boyardee rather than sectioning a fresh avocado that they're not paying any attention to what you're doing at all.

And if they are? If you meet someone with a seemingly perfectly pulled-together life and it turns out that you're right: She is totally judging you and thinking that you're a disgrace because you chose not to sleep-train/still let your son use a pacifier/don't always get a comb through your daughter's hair/wear mismatched socks? You do not want to be friends with that person.

Neither do I.

And I don't *have* to be friends with them. Neither do you. Isn't that a relief?

It's a choice, and nowadays I choose to opt out of the who's-a-better-parent merry-go-round: I just want to put caffeine in my body and get to know someone, and so that's what I try to do. It's so easy to get caught up in the web of judgment . . . but frankly, it's a huge waste of time, and chances are you don't have a ton of extra time lying around to waste. And as it turns out, the people that you make the effort to connect with are more often than not wonderful and interesting and comforting and empathetic and thoughtful and kind and *human.*

Choosing to be positive, to seek out interaction, to keep trying to forge relationships in a world where true friendship can sometimes feel in short supply . . . it's not only worth the work, it actually takes far less energy than wading through all that loneliness and fear.

More to the point, though: It's a hell of a lot more fun.

How-To: MAKE BUDDIES WHO HAVE BABIES

USE YOUR KIDS. Mommy and Me classes are just super-cute, and a great way to meet parents with similar interests (whether that's swimming, music, art, or dance) and kids the same age as your own. The first winter that we spent in our new town I signed up for a music class and a gym class with my son, and it was the best: We got out of the house, had fun together, and ended up making wonderful friends who stayed in our lives long after the courses came to an end.

JUST SAY YES. Even if you're not a "joiner" (I'm not either), this is a great time to accept any and all invitations. Help out with a bake sale? Absolutely. Come over for a playdate? Sure. Go to a yoga class? Why yes, I would love to.

LET IT GO. Just like in junior high, sometimes friendships don't work out. Not everyone will respond warmly to an offer of friendship; not everyone will like your kid and want your kid to hang out with their kid; not everyone will have space in their life for a new relationship. That's just the way it goes, and it's okay. You almost certainly did nothing "wrong," and wondering what happened is a waste of time and energy.

BE PATIENT. Remember the first week of freshman year of college? You met something like thirty-six thousand people, and then eventually sorted through them all until you were left with the handful of kindred spirits with whom you developed lasting friendships. Making for-real friends is no easy feat; it's a process that takes time and patience.

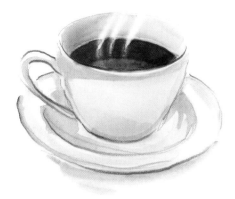

Conclusion

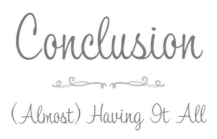

(Almost) Having It All

Did you know, one of my least favorite expressions on the planet is "having it all"? I suspect that the goal of the phrase is to inspire . . . but to me, it seems like what it actually does is undermine, implying that unless a woman can do everything perfectly, unless she can achieve it "all" (whatever "all" is), something is missing. The focus turns to what one is lacking, rather than what one has. And of course what each woman wants and does not want from her life is a hugely individual thing, so the very concept by nature breeds discontent, competition, and a pervasive sense of inadequacy.

Inadequacy is a terrible feeling; I know this from vast personal experience. When you feel like you're not good enough, it's hard to feel joyful . . . and the joy is what matters.

I do not want you to feel like you should "have it all."

I don't even know what "having it all" *means*.

"But Jordan!" you say, "that expression is in the title of your book! Did you make a fairly major typo?"

Let me tell you a little story about my very first car. (I'm going somewhere with this, I promise.)

My first car was a white Chrysler LeBaron convertible with a red velvet interior. I bought it from my aunt during my senior year of college, and drove it cross-country with my dad and my stuff a few weeks later.

Now, look: I'm just not the most conscientious car owner in the world, and this rather unlovely quality of mine was especially prominent in my early twenties. The front passenger seat of my LeBaron was usually filled with things like Carl's Jr. bags and old audition scripts, the front hubcaps were completely different from the back ones thanks to an odd hubcap-pilfering incident in a Vegas parking lot, the airbags were missing because I once hit another car with my car and couldn't afford to get them replaced, so I just cut them out using a pair of nail scissors and patched them with some duct tape, and I may have once forgotten to change the oil for two years (this, as it turns out, is a rather poor idea).

By the time that the car died (and it really did die; I had to call the guys who deal with actual deceased cars to haul it off of the curb in front of my house), it wasn't what anyone would have considered a beauty queen. Still: beauty queen or no, I loved it *so much*. I thought it was the coolest-looking car I'd ever seen. I lived in the land of Range Rovers and Lamborghinis, and I suspect very strongly that no one who saw me rolling down the street was awestruck by my car's amazingness quite as much as I was, but honestly: I didn't care what anyone else thought about it.

I didn't love my car because other people said it was cool; I loved it because when I rolled down the top I could feel the sun shining on my arms, because it was exactly the kind of car I'd always dreamed I'd drive up and down the PCH one day, and because it was *a white convertible with red velvet seats*. I mean, come on. That's pretty cool.

More than anything, though, was this: It was a car for that life that I was living right then, Carl's Jr. bags, old audition scripts and all. It made sense to me. It made me happy even during times when not a whole lot else did.

You know what kind of car I want today? A station wagon. One that's safe and gets decent mileage, and that I can throw my dogs and kid into and go wherever and feel reasonably certain that we're all going to get there happy and in one piece. We currently own a 2006 Subaru Outback: I think there are strawberry stains on the backseat, and my dogs have utterly destroyed the trunk, and I really don't care. The car is also blue, and I don't love blue cars, but when we went to the used car lot it was the one that was in the best shape within our price range, and guess what else I love these days? Cars that are in good shape and within my price range. I want functioning airbags, not duct-taped ones. I still want red velvet seats, but alas, Subaru Outbacks don't appear to come with that particular option.

The fact is, what you need and what you want out of life doesn't always stand still over time. I used to love having a tiny, elegant espresso sofa; now I want a big, smooshy couch boat. Things change. That's why it doesn't matter what some style expert or another says you should want; what matters is what *you* want. Sometimes a little luxury can do wonders for your sanity . . . and other times you don't give a snack pack about things like pre-heated seats and moon roofs; you just want to get there *now*, and without any more yelling, please.

You don't need to make sure that all your bases are covered and your check marks checked and your choices pre-approved by whoever hands down the grades for grown-up achievements. You need to be straight with yourself about what makes you happy (and even about those things that you secretly desire even though you might be too afraid to even say the words out loud), and then do your best not only to make those things happen, but to take it easy on yourself when they "almost" do . . . but then don't.

"Almost" is okay. Great, even.

Parenthood forces you to find ways to get more creative than you ever felt possible, and now you get to use that creativity to find ways—perhaps small, abbreviated ones—to make the things that you love a part of your life. That's something that I think I suspected way back when I was wearing ball gowns to chemistry class and getting my glitter eye shadow on, but that hit home a whole lot harder on the sunny October morning when my son arrived and showed me that when it comes down to it, lists are only so much paper. Checking everything off isn't the endgame. It's not even close to the point.

The point is to weave in what you love in the ways that work for you.

It's just like they told me in my ninth-grade acting class: Improvisation is everything.

Epilogue

Before my son was born I was never around kids much. I wouldn't say that I didn't "like" them, but I certainly didn't get all misty-eyed about them. When people handed their children to me I'd hold them for exactly the amount of time that felt "not rude" . . . and then hand them right on back.

Truth? I was a little nervous about becoming a mother . . . but I sort of operated on the expectation that I'd love my son and love being with him because you love your child and that is that.

And then, just like everyone tells you is going to happen, my son was born and there was the Before in my life, and the After. I cringe when I hear people say things like "You never know love until you're a mother"—because oof, the patronizing, oof, the self-righteousness—and I do not think that's true for everyone. I think people who choose not to or can't have children for whatever reason are capable of love just as great and deep as those who do or can.

But for me, for me personally? This is not a love that I knew existed.

I wake up in the middle of the night sometimes and let myself into his room and stand there, watching my son sleep and just missing him. Wishing it was morning already. Crying about it sometimes, and waking my husband up to ask him if our son is happy, if he is okay, if he knows how much we love him. And then the sun rises and alarms go off, jackets must be put on, and dogs must be ushered out for a walk. I'm much saner now that the light is back and coffee has been drunk, and when I start having to answer emails or take phone calls or sit down and write, I go ahead and let my son play on his own for a bit while I get things done, because he is fine and I have to do the things that I have to do and such is life.

And then night falls again, and the missing starts again, and I think back on my day and my heart aches with how badly I wish I could do it over, put down the phone or the computer and not cook or write or do anything at all (even though I love and want and need to cook and write and do thing after thing), just be with my baby before . . .

Before he—it, this, we—is gone.

In my Before days, when I told people that I really wasn't a "kid" person, I think it was just that I didn't see it. I wasn't paying attention to what's so bright and spectacular and beautiful about children: the wonder that's written right there across their faces when they see anything from a dog to a leaf to the fire trucks parked in the lot down the street. The other day I spent a solid thirty minutes opening and closing our car door because for some reason this made my son laugh hard enough that he nearly collapsed on the ground. I opened the door, then closed it, and watched him laugh. And then I did it again, and again, and again.

It's wonderful. Of course it is.

And it *hurts*.

Because love like this—for me, anyway—comes hand-in-hand with fear. I don't know how it is for everyone—and I've always been jealous of those people who can exist in the moment and feel grateful that it exists at all rather than mourning its loss even as it's happening—but to me, Real Love is a scary thing.

I'm scared for all the things that can happen, from actual, for-real dangers to the much more abstract sadness associated with aging out of the time when pure joy can be found in things like slides and bathtub ducks. Sometimes it feels like even the most mundane moments with my son (taking a bite, turning a page, petting a dog) are filled with the kind of excitement and beauty that in my former life was reserved for rare and glorious occasions like, say, falling in love for the first time, or graduating high school, or getting a dream job . . . and so when even the littlest of times moves into history, it slams into me with all the force of the passing of one of Life's Great Events.

I've said before how crazy it makes me, the constant reminders from everyone in the world who sees you holding your baby that "it goes too fast." And I think what I've come to realize now is that it makes me crazy because it's true, and they're right, and now that my son is running and laughing and talking, things are speeding up at a breakneck pace.

I just want to hold on to every single second, that's all. See everything, when of course not everything can be seen.

And of course the reality is that even if it lasted fifty years, the experience of raising our children would feel too short. Our nostalgia for our babies' fleeting childhood is sewn right up with nostalgia for our own, with our own memories of being held by parents who are too far away, these days. Who we wish would stroke our foreheads like they used to. And so we stroke our own children's foreheads, and it makes us feel better for the moment even as we're all too aware that that moment will pass.

I don't want it to go, that's all. But it will, and it should, and it must, and the alternative—to not build beautiful memories—is of course no alternative at all, and so one last lesson to be learned in Grown-up World, it seems, is to live in and with and for what's happening right now, rather than pushing forward into the After before it's even arrived. It's true: That After might be different in ways that you wish it weren't, but it will also be filled with adventures that you never saw coming. Because if there's one thing that motherhood has taught me, it's that life likes to throw a surprise or two your way.

I mean, like I said: I didn't know that love like this existed at all, and now I do.

Who knows what I'll know next?

Acknowledgments

First and foremost, thank you to the Ramshackle Glam readers— especially those who were there at the way, way beginning and came along for the ride while I figured a few things out (and then a few more). Thank you for being patient with my missteps along the way and thoughtful with your comments, and for helping to create a community that makes every single one of my days better and brighter.

Mom and Dad, your belief that the best place for a child to grow up is on the back of a motorcycle with a book in her hand is possibly the greatest gift I've ever been given. Thank you for showing me what it means to be your weird, wonderful self; I love you both (very much).

Thank you from the bottom of my heart to the amazing team at Digital Brand Architects, and especially to Karen Robinovitz, Reesa Lake, Kendra Bracken-Ferguson, Raina Penchansky, Vanessa Flaherty, Laura Minch, and Netta Ruth: You gave me confidence when I needed it the most, made me believe in possibilities far beyond my wildest dreams, and push me to do better every single day. Thank you also to Deborah Schneider at Gelfman Schneider for your guidance and encouragement (and for taking a chance).

To my editor, Cindy De La Hoz, and the phenomenal publishing team at Running Press, especially Amanda Richmond, Frances SooPingChow, Susan Hom, Jordana Tusman, Stacy Schuck, Chris Navratil, and Allison Devlin: Thank you for your generous support and hard work helping this book come together. It's been an honor working with you.

Debbie Mintcheff, thank you for your eagle-eye with all those recipes, and for getting me interested in food in the first place way back when.

Katie Rodgers, thank you for the privilege of lending your extraordinary talent to my book.

Enormous thank-yous also go to my wonderful parents-in-law, Tom and Lynn (and the whole Strauch family) for their love and constant belief that where we were headed was somewhere good; Naava Katz for the beautiful Ramshackle Glam logo; Nina Shield for handing me the match; Koa Beck and Eve Vawter at Mommyish.com for the daily dose of sanity and laughter (and for making the phrase "I don't give a snack pack" part of my world); the Reid family for showing me that you can sing if you want to; Todd Goldstein for the graphics advice (and the writing soundtrack); Julia Allison for making me sit down and write that very first blog post; Marianne Mancusi, Seth Feldman, and John Houghton for helping me discover what I loved to do; Penny Herbert for the many, many weekend trips; Stephen and Dave for the rooftop chats; Paige and Nadine for keeping me company on the sunny side; the wonderful people at the YMCA for helping us feel like we'd found not just a place to live, but a home; and Katie Kornstein for showing me that sometimes nothing works quite as well as a chill pill.

Morgan, my mama soul mate: Thank you for your early readings and your thoughtful notes, and for always being there, no matter what. You are an inspiration every single day.

Thank you to Ella for being a second pair of eyes both for my book and for my son; you are a part of our family forever.

I always wanted a sister, but never suspected she'd show up when I was twenty-five years old and sitting in a sushi restaurant whining about my sunburned back. Francesca, thank you for never for one second letting up on your insistence that I should do a crazy thing like be a writer, for being a touchstone of kindness and wisdom in good times and bad, and for showing me what true friendship is all about.

Kendrick, six years ago I stood in front of our family and friends and told you that I gave you my heart to hold in your hands. In return you gave me yours, and then you gave me our beautiful son, and I want you to know that you hold my heart still. Thank you for your kindness, for your patience, and for your unwavering faith in what could be.

Finally, for River: Everything. The whole world, if you want it.

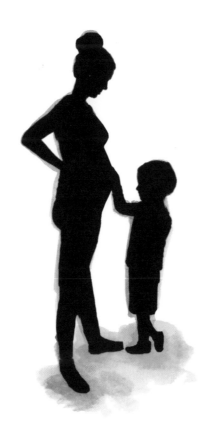